Magic for Lovers

The Wiccan Way to Lasting Romance

Selene Silverwind

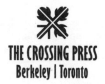

THE CROSSING PRESS
Berkeley | Toronto

To Brian,
for the romance that inspired this book.

To Brighid & Ogmios,
for giving me the inspiration and the words.

To my parents,
for showing me that love can last a lifetime.

The Crossing Press
A Division of Ten Speed Press
PO Box 7123
Berkeley CA 94707
www.tenspeed.com

Crossing Press titles are distributed in Australia by Simon & Schuster Australia, in Canada by Ten Speed Canada, in the United Kingdom and Europe by Airlift Books, in South Africa by Real Books, and in New Zealand by Southern Publishers Group.

Cover design by Wilsted & Taylor
Text design by Betsy Stromberg

ISBN 1-58091-152-8

Library of Congress Cataloging-in-Publication Data available from the publisher.

Printed in the United States

1 2 3 4 5 6 — 09 08 07 06 05 04

Grateful acknowledgement is made to Jeffrey Tye for permission to reprint "The Yoni Massage" ©1995, 2001 appearing on pages 135–38 and for "The Lingam Massage" ©1995, 2001 appearing on pages 138–41.

Table of Contents

PART TWO: ENHANCING RITUALS & BLESSINGS

PART THREE: UNITING CEREMONIES & BLESSINGS

PART FOUR: HEALING & BANISHING RITUALS

Contents

PART FIVE: BLESSINGS & MANIFESTING RITUALS

APPENDICES

BEFORE YOU BEGIN . . .

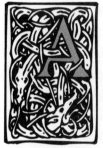ll too often our wedding day is the first and last time we manifest the spiritual aspects of our primary romantic relationship. We are married by a priest or priestess, we state our vows in a religious setting, such as a church or temple, and we include prayers and blessings throughout the event. However, as soon as the ceremony ends, this special spiritual experience is replaced with the mundane details of daily life and relegated to the obscurity of a photo album or video.

I believe spirituality should be the foundation of your relationship and play an active role in assuring its longevity. If you need a little help adding more soul *and* more sizzle to your life, you've come to the right place. *Magic for Lovers* offers dozens of rituals that can help you re-ignite passion, strengthen your bond as a couple, help you work through the tough times, and aid you in manifesting your long-term goals. It will also remind you to cherish each other every single day.

Throughout the text I use the term *lover,* rather than *partner, husband, wife, boyfriend, girlfriend, mate, spouse,* or *significant other.* I believe you should always think of your partner as your lover first and foremost, before all other titles, with the possible exception of *friend.* Calling your beloved by the word that is usually reserved for the bedroom serves as a constant reminder that the two of you love each other in a way that you love no one else.

Keep in mind that whenever you perform a ritual your *intention* is far more important than the actual words you say. And your words, no matter how simple, will be more effective if they come from your heart than if you read from a script that holds no meaning for you. My suggestions are intended to be just that: suggestions. Adapt them to suit your needs, your moods, your feelings.

If you make a mistake, feel free to laugh about it. Don't worry if the ritual isn't flawless. I don't think I've ever accomplished the perfect spell when more than one person was involved in it. And if all this is new to you, I recommend that you read through the book in sequence, then select the rituals when the mood strikes or the need arises.

Some of the metaphysical practices I mention throughout the book may not be familiar to you. What follows are very brief descriptions that I hope will inspire you to further study.

Feng Shui has come to be popularly thought of in the West as the Chinese art of furniture arrangement, but it's much, much more than that. This complex system for arranging your physical environment to maximize the positive flow of *qi* (pronounced "chee"), or the life force, employs two methods. I use the feng shui principles of the Black Hat method, which divides the home into nine equal sections, or *guas*. Each *gua* focuses on a different aspect of your life, and in this book, I will deal exclusively with the relationship and love *guas*.

Kundalini Yoga and the Seven Chakra System come to us from India. The chakras are energetic fields in and around the body that I like to imagine as spinning spheres of colored light. The first, or base, chakra at the bottom of your torso is red and relates to basic physical survival issues. The second chakra is orange and swirls around your sexual organs and its focus is, not surprisingly, centered on sexuality. The third chakra is yellow and located in the solar plexus, which is near the "v" below your ribs. Its focus is power. The heart chakra is green and influences love and relationships. The fifth chakra, also known as the communication chakra, is blue and resides in your throat. The sixth indigo-colored chakra, also referred to as the third eye, resides behind the center of your forehead and focuses on intuition and imagination. The seventh chakra is violet-colored and is the seat of your spirituality at the crown of your head.

If you are familiar with Hatha Yoga, the ancient practice of controlling your breath as you move through a series of postures, creating a union between body, mind, and breath, then you will already be comfortable with many of the techniques I recommend.

Tantra has been much in the media lately, largely due to celebrities extolling its sexual benefits, and made famous by the Kama Sutra, the ancient Indian text that describes various sexual positions, many of which require exceptional strength and flexibility. Tantric Yoga, however, is a complex system that incorporates

Kundalini Yoga, among many other techniques, for attuning and harnessing the sexual energy of your body and your lover's body to achieve transformation and transcendence. I have adapted only the most basic of those practices, and you should have no trouble mastering them.

The rituals in this book draw heavily on beliefs and practices common to **Wicca,** which is a branch of **Neo-Paganism.** Neo-Paganism is an umbrella term for several earth-based or recreated pre-Christian religions. Pagans worship deities that pre-date Jesus, Mohammed, and Buddha, although some Pagans adopt Buddhist practices or Christian figures into their faiths. Most Pagans honor deities and follow traditions from various ancient cultures, including Native American, Egyptian, Greek, Celtic, Germanic, Scandinavian, African, and South American.

Wiccans commonly worship both a god and a goddess, or multiple gods and goddesses. They follow the Wheel of the Year, or cycle of the seasons, the Rede, which states, "And it harm none, do what thou wilt," and the Law of Three, which states that whatever energy you release returns to you threefold. For these reasons, most Wiccans refrain from hexes or curses. Wiccan magic is a method of manipulating energy and the elements of earth, air, fire, water, and spirit to a desired end, which can be anything from world peace to a salary increase. Many Wiccan rituals and spells adhere to a basic common framework, which is what you will find in this book

A full understanding of each of these practices is not needed to use the spells and rituals that follow, but if you are interested in further study, the bibliography lists several useful references. For current links to suppliers for the products I mention, please visit my website, www.SeleneSilverwind.com.

Now, go to it! Enhance! Unite! Heal! Manifest! And above all, Love one another! May your days be filled with joy, abundance, love, and fabulous sex!

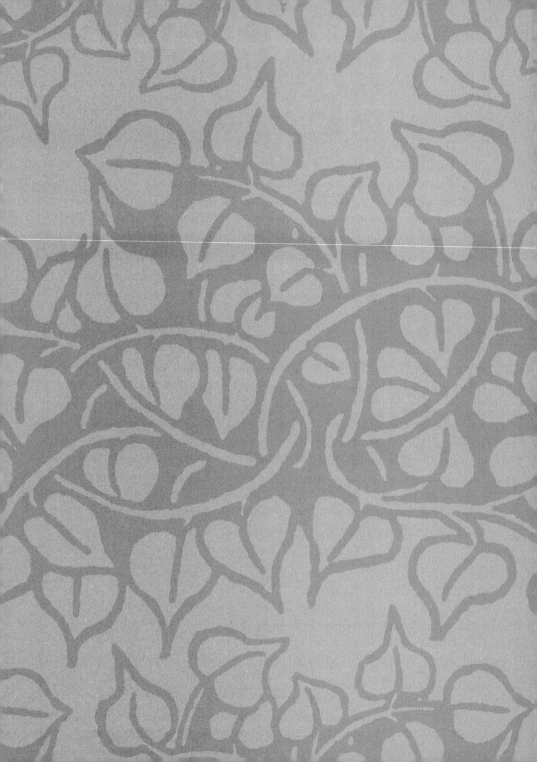

A FEW WORDS ABOUT LOVE & MAGIC

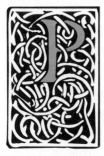eople are wired for love. It has been celebrated for centuries as a necessity of life, as something intrinsic to human nature. We encourage love in all its many forms, such as parental love, platonic love, agape love, and romantic love.

I seem to be have been gifted with intuitive insights into love, and I'm happy to share my gifts with others. I prefer to offer spells, rituals, or advice that is non-manipulative in nature, but from time to time I meet those who are so desperate they will risk the repercussions of unethical uses of magic.

Because my background is Wiccan, I attempt to follow the Wiccan Rede, which is to harm no one. However, love has many gray areas, so through study, meditation, and experience, I have developed some ground rules regarding what I will and will not do:

I will never perform a spell designed to attract a specific person.

Imagine that Sheryl has met the man of her dreams. She just knows it was meant to be, but her interest isn't returned. She dresses just so, hangs around him as much as possible, and drops little hints, and still nothing. She knows in her heart that he just needs a little nudge. So she casts a spell. An innocent spell to attract him to her. She's in love, so what's the harm in making her heart's desire return her affection?

Suddenly, he calls every day, asks her out, and wants to be her boyfriend. Great! It worked. The two of them are encased in a magic bubble. They spend all their time together. They don't need anyone or anything except each other. Their lives are perfect.

Or are they? Their jobs are in trouble because they frequently come in late, or leave early, or don't come in at all because they can't bear to be apart. Their friends have given up on them. Neither can bear to see the other speaking to someone else of the opposite sex.

See anything wrong with this picture? Think it sounds farfetched? Think again. It is a classic co-dependent relationship, and it's the best you can hope for when you cast a spell to "make" someone love you. There is a reason why.

Many Pagans believe in some form of karma or a law of return, the idea being that the energy you release into the world returns to you like a boomerang. In some traditions the return is threefold in its intensity. This isn't simply a magical theory. As we know from physics: for every action, there is an equal and opposite reaction. In magical terms, energy can be unpredictable, regardless of how experienced the practitioner is. Thus, spells can sometimes have unexpected or unwelcome consequences.

But if it's love energy, what could be wrong with that?

A lot, because love energy is extremely powerful. You risk becoming obsessed with your beloved and you risk becoming an object of obsession yourself. Although this might seem flattering at first, it won't for long. *Obsession is not the same as love.*

When you try to "make" someone love you, you are manipulating their will. You're forcing them to do something they might not otherwise do. This is a form of psychic rape. Rape, in any form, is a violation, no matter what your intentions. And do you really want someone to love you because you "made" them do it? Will you ever be able to really trust those feelings? Probably not.

Finally, spells don't last forever. How long a spell will last depends on your specifications when performing it. Magical energy typically weakens after a season (three months) has passed. Manipulative spells doom the relationship to ultimate failure. Because the feelings were forced in the first place, rather than allowed to develop naturally, when the spell wears off, the feelings will evaporate too, causing you much heartbreak.

What can you do when you're attracted to someone and hope to catch his or her eye? Do the same things everyone else does. Call and ask for a lunch date or a night at the movies. Develop a closer friendship. Show off your best qualities. You don't need magic to make these things happen. If you think you need magical assistance, cast a spell to make *yourself* feel more attractive and confident and communicative.

If you're not pining for someone specific, but do want to draw love into your life, make a list of qualities your ideal lover would possess and cast a spell to attract someone with those qualities. This isn't manipulation because you're not saying, "You, over there, in the green shirt, with the blue eyes, named Jason. You will love me, starting now." You are saying, "Whoever is the right person, please come to me."

I will never perform a love spell on behalf of someone else.

I've been asked many times to cast love spells for other people, either because they didn't feel they had the skill to do it themselves, or because they wanted an "expert" to do it for them.

You don't have to be a professional or possess special powers for magic to be effective. Remember, it's your intention that counts, not your level of expertise. Instead of casting spells *for* people, I explain how to do the spells themselves. I have four reasons for this policy: First, to be sure the spell works only on your friend and not you, you must place restrictions on it that could cancel out the spell's energy entirely. Second, despite your best efforts, you could be ensnared by the spell anyway. Third, and perhaps most obviously, love spells are most effective when performed by the person asking for love.

And finally, when you cast a love spell, you're sending your energy out into the universe and the universe is looking for a match to that energy. Casting the spell for a friend might draw love into *your* life instead of the intended target's!

This rule applies not only to love attraction spells, but also to spells performed on behalf of someone you love. Although this may seem like an ethical gray area, I don't see it that way. Even if you think someone you care about needs your help, if you have not been asked, don't perform the spell. You may not know the entire story, and your well-meaning attempts to help may actually worsen the situation.

It is very painful to watch your loved ones harm themselves, but you don't have the right to magically interfere until you're asked. We all have lessons we need to learn in life, and interference could prevent that lesson from being learned, or even prolong the suffering, which you certainly wouldn't wish!

When doing spell work, especially when it involves love or people you love, you must consider *all* the possible results. What seems helpful might actually cause more harm in the end. If you're asked to cast a spell for someone else, I advise you to give advice or provide information instead. Avoid doing the magic for them.

I never magically interfere in someone else's relationship.

Often I'm asked to interfere with or break up relationships. For instance, one young man asked me to break up his sister and her girlfriend because he believed they were sinning. Another young man asked me to break up a couple so he could date the young woman himself.

Of course, I said no in both cases. In the first, I felt that if the two women had found love with each other, then the relationship was right for them. In the second, the would-be suitor was free to intervene using non-magical methods—without my help. For magic to be effective, it must be backed up by belief, will, intent, and right. Magic doesn't work if you don't have the guts to take a simultaneous action in the real world. If you choose magic because you aren't comfortable taking the same action through more traditional means, then you shouldn't be using magic at all. Such last resort uses of magic are unethical to my way of thinking.

But you don't have to sit on your hands when you sense a problem, particularly if physical abuse, substance abuse, or other destructive behavior has entered the picture. You are certainly free to express your opinions or recommend counseling or both.

It is also tempting to use magic to "save" a marriage that's in trouble, especially if you're close to the couple. Don't. You're not in the relationship. Don't make it your karma.

 I never perform a spell on my lover without his or her permission.

I'm always asked, "Why not?" It's simple. It's a matter of trust. Trust is the most important aspect of any relationship. If you feel you must cast a spell behind your lover's back, then your relationship is already in big trouble. It is manipulative. You are lying. Neither is a sign of a healthy relationship. Furthermore, if you feel compelled to lie to or manipulate your lover, regardless of how "loving" your intentions, then you should probably ask yourself, "Why?" instead of "Why not?" If you can't tell your lover your plans, you probably already know the answer. Would you like it if your lover ignored your feelings and manipulated you? You would not. So give your lover the same consideration you would expect for yourself.

A secret spell may provide a quick fix for the difficulty you're experiencing, but it can't provide a long-term solution because the issues at the heart of the problem have not been dealt with. The problem will simply continue to resurface.

A common misuse of love magic occurs during a romantic or sexual dry spell, which many couples experience from time to time. People are complicated, and they bring their complications into their relationships, and often into the bedroom. Rather than resorting to manipulation as your first line of defense, try a little self-evaluation. Is it really all your lover's fault? Or could some of the issues possibly come from you?

Use your magical tools on yourself instead of your lover. Enhancing rituals will help you open your mind and your heart to whatever your lover has to offer. Healing rituals will help you release any pain or anger or resentment that could be coming between you and your lover. Cleansing rituals will help purify your home of lingering, energy-sapping negativity. Uniting and renewing rituals will help you return to that common ground you never thought you'd lose.

Often, I'm asked how to perform a relationship spell if the person's lover doesn't "believe in" magic. If this is your situation, do you what you can by yourself to cleanse and bless your home, boost your self-esteem and self-confidence, rid yourself of stress and negativity, and improve your communication skills. Explain to your lover how important a certain ritual is to you.

Merging differing faiths is one of the challenges many Pagans face. Most important is that you and your lover respect each other's faiths, whatever they may be. Try to share them whenever you can. Perhaps you could attend your lover's synagogue on a high holiday. Maybe your lover would participate in a gratitude ritual with you.

Be open-minded. Be flexible. I know devout Christians who have successful relationships with Pagans. As long as there is mutual respect, you should be fine. If problems do arise, communication is the key. Although shared experiences will help strengthen the bond between you, give each other plenty of space.

Even within Paganism, there are many differing traditions and you and your lover may not share the same one. Together you can create unique spells just for the two of you. Consider writing a relationship dedication that draws on the deities and practices of both your traditions. Place symbols from both faiths on a relationship altar. Celebrate the holidays by merging some rituals. While certain deities don't like to be called together, if they're your personal deities, then I don't think they'll mind. If they do, find another deity to watch over your relationship.

Even when we use our best intentions, sometimes love and magic can become muddled. I've codified these "rules" as a guide to help you find your own way into a successful merger of love and magic. Ask yourself the following before using magic on someone you love:

- ❦ *Am I attempting to manipulate the will of another person?*
- ❦ *Would I be willing to cause my desired result without using magic?*

❦ *What are all the possible results and repercussions?*

❦ *Has my intended target asked me to the cast this spell?*

By the time you get to the fourth question, you will know whether or not the spell is appropriate. When in doubt, use your common sense.

All the spells in this book have been written for you and your lover together, so manipulation is not a worry when using them. Let this chapter serve as your guide when creating spells on your own.

Part One

Tools &
Techniques

What follows are items and practices you will use over and over again for many, if not most of the rituals, spells, and ceremonies in this book. Of course, don't be afraid to be creative and let your imagination supplement these suggestions.

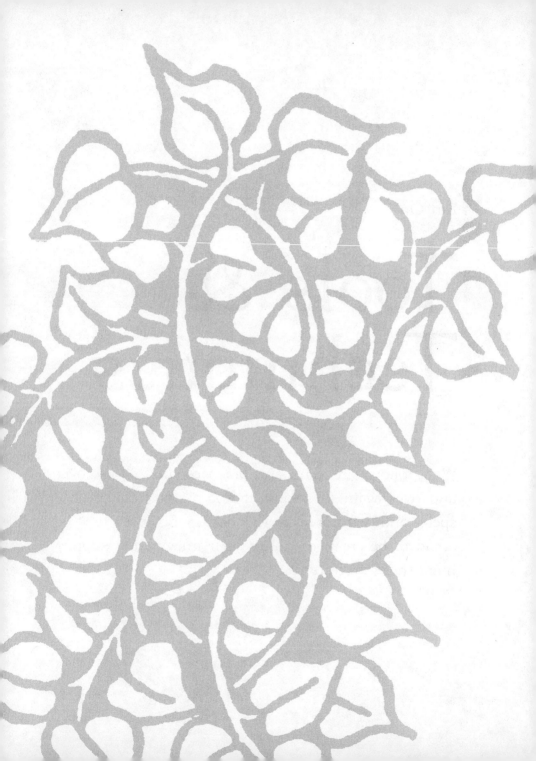

Chapter 1

BEDROOM FENG SHUI

o book about romantic rituals would be complete without a discussion of bedroom feng shui. (See page viii for a brief description of feng shui basics.)

Draw the love symbol (see below) on parchment paper and place it under your bed or between the mattress and box spring to ensure that your bedroom will be a safe haven for romance and love. If you are in a same-sex relationship, adapt the symbol accordingly.

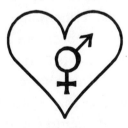

The Love Symbol

If you have a special occasion planned, put red sheets on the bed. Satin will probably feel fantastic, but slippery sheets and active lovemaking may not mix well. Make sure your sheets, including your everyday sets, have a high thread count. They will they last longer and make your bed that much more inviting. I use 250-thread cotton sheets. Talk about luxurious!

The scents of lavender and roses send a cue to the brain that romance beckons. Sprinkle lavender or rose water on the bed, place a sachet of lavender and roses near or under the bed, or sprinkle the sheets with lavender or rose-scented powder. Be careful. Too much fragrance can be overpowering. And there's nothing sexy about a sneezing fit. At least once, make love on a bed of rose petals. Not because it's a feng shui concept, but just because it's fun.

Your bedroom is for sex, sleeping, and laughter. It is not a bastion of seriousness. It is a sensual haven for love and sensuality and continuous reconnection with your lover. Ban the television and computer from the bedroom. They draw attention away from what should be the focus of this very special room, they interfere with sleep, and they inhibit lovemaking.

In feng shui terms, the area of your bedroom you should most concentrate on is the relationship corner. To find this area, stand in the doorway of your bedroom and look to the far right corner. In your mind's eye, extend that corner out to create a square that is a ninth of the room's size. This is your relationship corner. If you have any oddly shaped walls here, imagine that the area extends to the outside to make a square. You may want to hang a round, faceted crystal from the ceiling to deflect energy away from any sharp corners jutting into the room from this area. When possible, place your love altar (see page 27), in this corner of the bedroom.

Every room in your home has a relationship corner, as does your entire living space. To find the relationship corner of your home, stand in your front doorway and look to the far right corner of the structure. Again, extend this area out in your mind's eye to comprise an area the equivalent of a ninth of your living space. This is your home's relationship corner. Mine falls in the area of my kitchen where I store cooking equipment and leave my dishes to dry. To correct the energy of the area, I put a piece of red silk in one of the cupboards. It energizes this area of my home and my relationship. If your home's relationship corner falls in an awkward spot, try something similar.

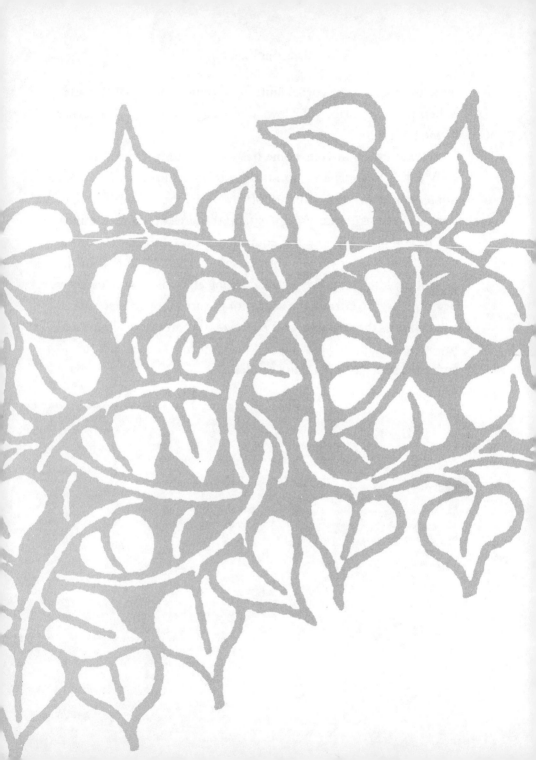

Chapter 2

LOVE OIL

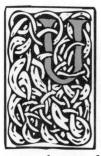se love oil with an aromatherapy burner to scent the room, rub into pressure points on your lover's body, apply to candles, or add to your potpourri. If you wish to bless your candles, as I do, there is a special technique for applying the oil for magical purposes. Place the oil on your fingertips, then rub it from the top of the candle down to the middle and from the bottom up to the middle. In this way, you draw love energy into your life and into the ritual.

You can make your own oil, have a local aromatherapist blend it for you, or purchase it already blended. (Individual oils can be found at New Age stores, natural food stores, aromatherapy stores, or online.) High quality is essential when blending the oils for love rituals. If you skimp on quality, it sends a message to the universe that you don't think your relationship is worth the expense.

Oils are best blended and stored in a dark green or amber glass bottle to prevent evaporation and corruption from ambient light. Essential oils often come in bottles with droppers; otherwise use an eyedropper, rinsing it out with water after each oil is added.

Love Oil Blend

1 ounce almond or jojoba oil as a base
1 drop rose otto or absolute (pure, non-synthetic and non-blended oils)
1 drop rosemary oil
2 drops lavender oil
1 drop jasmine oil
2 drops ylang-ylang oil
2 drops rosewood oil

Pour the almond or jojoba base into the bottle first, then add the other oils. Swirl to mix. The scent of the blended oil will intensify over time. Store all your oils in a cool, dry place.

Note: High quality rose and jasmine oils are expensive, and worth it. If cost is a factor, rather than substituting with poor quality oils, you may use rose petals or jasmine flowers instead.

Chapter 3

LOVE BODY WASH

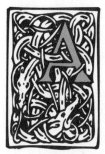 body wash is suggested for several of the healing rituals. Or use it to prepare for any ritual during your pre-ritual bath, which I highly recommend. A pre-ritual bath helps release your mind from mundane cares, and it signals your brain that you are about to do something special. Just pour a small amount onto a bath puff and bathe as usual.

Body Wash Blend

8 ounces unscented body wash base
1 drop rose otto or absolute
1 drop jasmine oil
2 drops rosewood oil
2 drops ylang-ylang oil
1 drop rosemary oil

This recipe is slightly different from the love oil, in which you added your essential oils to a base. Here, blend the oils together, then add them to an unscented body wash or shower gel. (You can find a body wash base at a beauty supply store or online.)

Chapter 4

COMFORTING

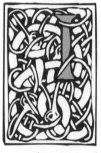n many ways, comforting is more important to your relationship than sex. Comforting helps you reconnect as a couple and heals any wounds between you, old and new. It also helps you show your support when your lover is suffering from a hardship or just feeling down.

My lover and I consider comforting one another a sacred duty. When I tell my lover I need comforting, he drops whatever he is doing and takes me into his arms, holding me and gently caressing me until I feel better. I do the same for him when he is in need of my support.

I recommend comforting in bed where you have the benefit of full-body contact, but it can be done anywhere. It doesn't have to be a marathon session, just long enough to reassure the one in need of comfort. You and your lover should agree that a comforting request will *always* be granted without question, even if it's

3 A.M. and you're in the middle of a juicy dream. I know this can be a challenge. I'm not a morning person, but my relationship is more important than ten minutes of extra sleep.

It is especially important to comfort one another after a fight or misunderstanding. I begin by saying "I'm sorry," whether or not I feel I was in the wrong. Even when I "know" I'm right, I'm *always* sorry our discussion became a fight. Making this statement shows my lover that I am willing to work out our differences and am dedicated to making our relationship work. After we've each apologized, we come together in whichever position we prefer and comfort each other until the hurt has dissipated.

We never go to sleep without cuddling or comforting, even if it's just for five minutes or over the phone. How do you cuddle over the phone? When my lover and I are apart for the night, we call to say goodnight and "I love you" after we've climbed into bed. These few moments of relaxed conversation remind us of our connection before we go to sleep.

There are no hard and fast rules for comforting. Allow your practice to evolve naturally and this will be the right way to comfort and be comforted. Every night, it is important to revel in the love you share. This small gesture will keep the spark more glowingly alive than you can possibly imagine.

Chapter 5

COUPLE-BREATHING

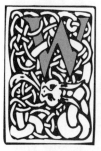

We all know that without breath there is no life, but I'm not referring to the involuntary act of breathing. I'm referring to a form of conscious breathing: breathing in unison, or shared breath. I call it couple-breathing, and I have found this technique to be especially powerful during rituals, as well as an incredible addition to lovemaking.

First, set the stage in the bedroom: clean sheets, peace and quiet, and lots of candles. Make sure you will be alone and won't be interrupted. Avoid wearing perfume or other intrusive scents. I also recommend not playing music; your breathing should be the only sound in the room.

Now undress each other and go to your bed or a soft rug on the floor. Sit comfortably cross-legged facing one another, knees touching, holding hands loosely. Close your eyes. Begin breathing, slowly. First, focus on your own breath. Don't force it. Just observe it. Relax. Let your breath slow naturally.

Once your breathing has become slow and even, listen to your lover's breath. Slowly adjust your breath (without causing yourself to hiccup) until you and your lover are exhaling and inhaling at the same time. Try to lengthen each breath you take together. Then, try to breathe more deeply in unison. Listen to the cues from your lover. Experiment. Try shallow breathing, deep breathing, breathing as you lie side-by-side, breathing while standing up body-to-body.

You can also share your breath by inhaling while your lover exhales so that you are breathing in a continuous cycle. Imagine that the breath travels down through your body, out through your lowest chakra, then travels up your lover's body, and creates a continuous flow of energy between you. Don't be afraid if you feel silly at first. If you need to laugh, go ahead. There is no right or wrong.

Couple-breathing can be tricky at first, but once you find your rhythm, it is amazing. It can be used as part of foreplay and can add an incredible intensity to intercourse, especially if you also include eye-gazing, that is, looking intently into other's eyes.

A more advanced maneuver involves breathing "through" different parts of the body. If you are familiar with yoga, you know what I mean. If not, this is how I do it: First, I focus on a particular part of my body. Then I inhale deeply, drawing the breath toward that body part. Let's start with your hands. Imagine your breath filling your hands. See if you can feel them expand with energy. Try to release any tension in them as you exhale.

Now place your hands against your lover's hands. Inhale, drawing your breathe in through your hands, drawing your lover's energy into you. Then exhale, allowing your lover to absorb your breath though his or her hands. Experiment with breathing into other parts of your body and see if the connection deepens.

There are many variations of couple-breathing, so don't be afraid to experiment and discover which method works for you. You will find it greatly enhances the relationship rituals you'll be using later in the book.

Chapter 6

EYE-GAZING

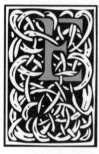ye-gazing is the simple act of looking lovingly into each others' eyes. Before you conjure up memories of childhood battles to see who could go the longest without blinking, let me clarify that eye-gazing is not a staring contest. It is not an attempt to catch each other in lies. It is not a chance to notice every line and wrinkle on your lover's face.

Eye-gazing helps bring you and your lover into synchronicity and enables you to see into each other's souls. It brings a new level of connection to your relationship, without spoken communication, and thus with less chance for misunderstanding. Eye-gazing can be added to any other ritual or technique in this book.

At first you might feel silly or uncomfortable. Try looking into your own eyes in the mirror. Take your time. Work up to it as a couple. If you need to look away, look away. If you need to giggle, giggle. When you are ready to gaze into each other's eyes again, do so for a little longer each time. Slowly but surely, you will become more comfortable.

Once you've become comfortable with eye-gazing, try adapting it to other practices. While practicing couple-breathing, look into your lover's eyes as you continue to breathe together. Feel free to blink. Feel free to smile. This is not a challenge. This is a loving exchange using only your breath and your eyes.

Try eye-gazing during lovemaking. It is truly an amazing experience to look into your lover's eyes as you reach orgasm—and vice versa. Although it may take some getting used to, it is an indescribably exciting and precious way for you and your lover to reveal yourselves to one another.

If eye-gazing during lovemaking and orgasm is too much for you at first, try adding a few minutes of eye-gazing to your foreplay. You will discover new dimensions to the emotional and spiritual connection between you.

Chapter 7

TANTRIC SITTING POSITION

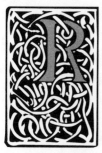eaders who are familiar with the principles and practice of Tantra won't be familiar with my name for this classic Tantric position. I've adapted it from what the Kama Sutra calls "Dolita," however, it is not Dolita in the strictest sense unless the practioners are engaged in intercourse. Because I use this position somewhat differently, I call it the "Tantric sitting position."

To move into the Tantric sitting position, my lover sits cross-legged on the floor or bed. I then sit facing him with my legs around his waist and my bottom in the space between his legs. Once in position, our eyes and lips are aligned and our chests, bellies, and genitals touch. (See the illustration on the following page.)

This position can be a part of fore-play or lovemaking, and it's a perfect position in which to practice couple-breathing and eye-gazing. I also love to comfort and be comforted in the Tantric sitting position. Because it brings your chakras into alignment, it is another way to deepen your connection during the energy-raising rituals.

The Tantric sitting position often leads to extremely pleasurable sex, because it allows you both to be fully aroused while placing your entire body within easy reach of lover for kissing and caressing—and vice versa. If you can, look into each other's eyes as you make love to more deeply experience the connection between you. Experiment with the Tantric sitting position and see where it leads you.

Chapter 8

CREATING SACRED SPACE

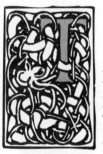he spells and rituals throughout this book are best performed within what I think of as "sacred space." There are two methods I use to create this: casting a circle and deep breathing. The first technique is more formal, more ritualized while the latter can be used in impromptu situations.

"Casting the circle" and "calling the quarters" are Wiccan techniques that delineate a circle of protective energy around you, your lover, and your ritual space. In addition to keeping negative energy out, it keeps the love energy you create within, allowing it to build on itself until you are ready to release it. These rituals also serve to cue your mind that you are about to do something special.

Calling the quarters means you are inviting the four elements and four directions to participate in the ritual. The quarters traditionally are: north/earth, east/air, south/fire, west/water. However, feel free to adjust the associations to your own surroundings. Always *invite* the elements, never command. These energies are stronger than you are, and they don't like being ordered around. Usually they will come when asked and willingly lend their energy to your ritual.

Before you cast the circle, clear the space where you will be performing the ritual. You may not be able to cast the circle all the way around your love altar or regular altar (see pages 27–29), in which case you can either set up a special altar somewhere else in the room or imagine the circle continuing all the way around the altar. You can also cast a circle around your entire bedroom if your ritual includes lovemaking, or around your entire home if you plan to visit more than one room during the ritual.

Casting the Circle & Calling the Quarters

You will need: a directional compass and one of the following— an athame, a wand, a rose, or simply your finger. (The traditional athame is a dull, double-sided ceremonial knife of any length. I've also used a decorative letter opener for this ritual.)

When you are ready to begin, follow these steps:

1. Use the compass to determine the directions, or guess as best you can by using the sun, stars, or local landmarks. Face in a generally northerly direction, although a precise position is not absolutely essential.

2. Stand up and move to the northern point of your circle. Holding your ritual object out in front of you, pointed

toward the floor, walk clockwise around your altar. (If you can't walk around it because of its placement, point with your ritual object or finger clockwise around the circle.) As you walk, repeat:

"Here lies the boundary of the sacred circle. Naught but love shall enter in. Naught but love shall emerge from within."

When you return to the northern point again, your circle is cast.*

3. Facing north, point your ritual object or finger in that direction, then say:

"Element of earth, spirits of the north, please join the sacred circle now and ground us in love."

Repeat this incantation for east/air, south/fire, west/water by using the following substitutions: for the east, ask air to inspire your hearts; for the south, ask fire to bring you passion; for the west, ask water to bless you with the emotion of love.

4. Now you are in the sacred circle.

* (Adapted from *Wicca: A Guide for the Solitary Practitioner* by Scott Cunningham.)

If you invite a deity or deities to join you, as recommended in the spells that follow, do so *after* you have called the quarters. Release any deities you've summoned *before* you release the quarters unless you are specifically asking a deity to remain. If you wish to invite the deity to remain, say: *"Stay if you will, go if you must. Farewell and blessed be."* (See Appendix D for a list of gods and goddesses.) If you feel uncomfortable inviting the gods and goddesses to join your ritual, feel free not to. However, I do recommend that you replace the specific deity names with God, Goddess, Universe, Higher Power, or whichever term feels right to you.

Releasing the Circle & Quarters

When you ready to conclude the ritual, follow these steps:

1. Start with the quarters, beginning in the west. Point your ritual object and say:

   "Element of water, spirits of the west, thank you for joining the sacred circle and blessing us with the emotion of love. Farewell and blessed be."

2. Release the other quarters by turning or walking counter-clockwise. Follow water with fire, then air, concluding with earth.

3. To open the circle, begin at the northern point and walk counter-clockwise around the circle, drawing the energy back into your ritual object, saying:

   "Here lay the boundary of the sacred circle. Naught but love entered in. Naught but love emerged from within. The circle is open but unbroken. Blessed be."

Deep Breathing

The alternative method to creating sacred space is something I call deep breathing, although it's really much more than that. First, you and your lover should clear the space where you will perform the ritual. Seat yourselves on the floor, bed, or in chairs with your knees touching. Reach out and hold hands. Now begin couple-breathing. You can eye-gaze or not. Slow your breathing, calm your mind, and open yourself up to the magical energies around you. When you are calm and quiet, begin by saying: *"We are now in sacred space."* Then continue with the ritual.

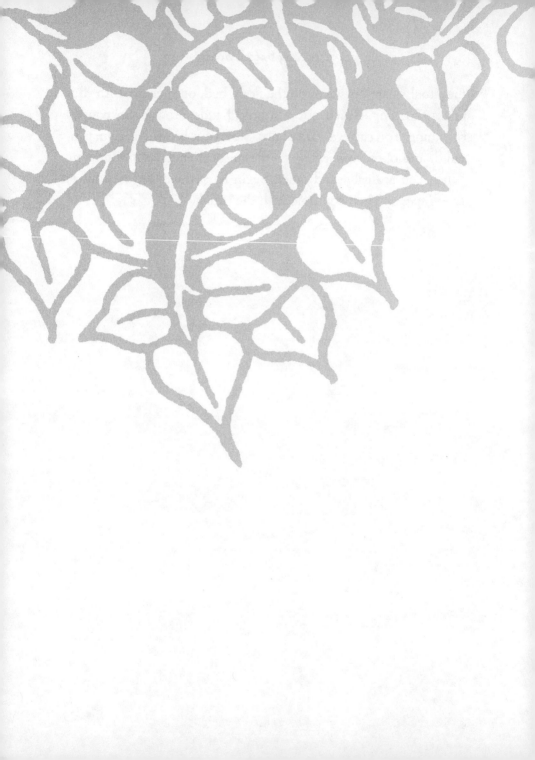

Chapter 9

THE LOVE ALTAR

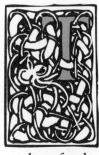he love altar is a tool for celebrating and enhancing the love that you share. It shows the gods that you and your lover are dedicated to each other and prompts them to give you a little help when you need it. Because it will be a focal point for many other rites and spells, I recommend performing this blessing ritual before moving on to the others.

My love altar is in the far right corner of my bedroom on a corner shelf I installed expressly for this purpose. Although my altar is too small to hold everything mentioned here, other items are arranged on a trunk below it. The altar itself is draped in a pink cloth, on top of which is a large pink candle on a small plate, a tiny statue of Aphrodite, a photo of my lover and myself, and a bowl filled with rose petals. The stuffed animals my lover has given me are also displayed on the trunk as a reminder of the special occasions we've shared.

Prior to performing the love altar blessing, you will need to find a suitable location for your altar and gather your altar adornments. The best place for your love altar is the relationship corner of your bedroom. If you absolutely cannot have your altar in your bedroom, choose the relationship area of your home.

The altar can be assembled on a wall shelf, a dresser, or a small table. You will need: an altar cloth (pink to represent romantic love, red to symbolize passionate love, or white for innocent love); a framed photo of you and your lover to help make your relationship the focus of the altar; a pink candle to bring fire to your relationship; a candleholder to catch drips and prevent accidents. The candle need not be lit at all times, but I recommend burning it at least fifteen minutes a week to recharge the energy in the room. A vase or bowl for flowers will represent the two of you as vessels of love. If you're using fresh flowers, be sure to replace them as soon as they start to wilt and change the water frequently. You may substitute petals or dried flowers from a bouquet that was a gift from one of you to the other. Rose quartz crystals on your altar will harness and amplify love energy. Prior to placing one on your love altar, cleanse it by soaking it in rock salt for three days or by leaving it outdoors under a full moon overnight.

If you wish to invite the protection or blessing of a deity into your relationship, place a statue of Aphrodite or another love goddess on your altar. If you want a romantic image, a reproduction of Rodin's "The Kiss" or a print of Klimt's "The Kiss" will draw passionate energy to your altar.

Lastly, small mementos from your first date, like movie stubs or a matchbook from the restaurant, complete your love altar.

You may keep objects from other rituals, such as handfasting cords or prosperity boxes, on your altar. Of course, there's no need to cram everything I've mentioned onto your altar. Only use what feels right to you.

Your altar should stay assembled at all times. Keep the photo current and the surface of the altar clean, orderly, and dust-free. A cluttered love altar can lead to a cluttered relationship. As you add new items to your altar, remove a few old ones to keep the relationship fresh.

Love Altar Blessing

You will need: a broom in addition to the items suggested above

When you and your lover are ready to bless your altar, follow these steps:

1. The altar surface should be in place, but bare. With your broom, symbolically sweep the area around the altar of any negative or clogged-up feelings. Sweep the corners of the ceiling too. There's no need to actually touch the surfaces, just imagine any negativity being swept away.

2. Cast the circle around your entire bedroom or wherever your altar is located. Invite the quarters and elements to join you.

3. Invite Aphrodite, or another female goddess, to attend your blessing:

   "Lady Aphrodite, goddess of love, passion, and romance, please join us as we build this altar as a testament to our

love. Bless it with your powers of love that it may keep the flame of our love burning for all time."

4. Decorate the altar by draping the pink cloth over it, add the framed photo, and say:

"We dedicate this altar to our love."

Set the pink candle in the holder in the middle of the altar. Light it and say:

"May our love burn as strongly as this flame."

Place the vase on the altar, saying:

"This is a vessel of love and a representation of us as vessels of love."

Add a rose to the vase, saying:

"May our love bloom as this flower blooms and never fade as the scent of a rose remains always sweet."

Place the crystal on your altar and say:

"This crystal is the physical manifestation of our love. May it amplify our love and encourage happiness."

5. The goddess statue should take a prominent place on the altar. Say:

"This statue serves as a reminder of your blessing. May it strengthen our love always."

If you are using another image, say:

"May it inspire our lovemaking for all time."

Add the remaining items you have selected. Be sure to include a blessing for the future with each one. For example, as you place the matches from your first dinner out together, say:

"May our lives be filled always with abundant sustenance."

6. When your altar is complete, join hands, eye-gaze, and couple-breathe. As you breathe together, feel the energy around you expanding to encompass the altar. Focus on infusing your altar with love. When you feel the energy has reached a high point, turn to the altar and say:

"This altar is a testament to our love. It is blessed with the powers of love so that it may keep the flame of our love burning for all time. So mote it be."

7. Thank Aphrodite for her blessing and release the quarters and circle. This is an ideal moment to make love to seal the altar blessing.

Chapter 10

SACRED SEX

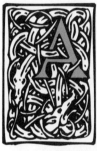

ll sex is sacred if it is undertaken with love, affection, and respect. When I refer to sacred sex, I mean sex that is deeper and performed for a greater purpose in addition physical pleasure.

You may conclude any of the rituals in this book with sacred sex. If you wish, you can create new sacred space around the bed before making love, or wait until after you have made love to release your existing sacred space.

I recommend making love in the Tantric sitting position or in any position that allows all of your chakras to be aligned. Connecting your chakras and your lover's chakras can be a part of foreplay. There's no need to rush to intercourse. Sacred sex can be slow, sensual, and purposeful. Delaying your orgasms for as long as possible can greatly heighten the energy. Extending the actual release for as long as you can will carry your intention to the gods.

After your orgasms, don't rush to separate your bodies. Often after sacred sex, I feel a bit dizzy or woozy from the intense energy that has been raised and released. Allow yourself time to recover before getting up to do other things. Let your intuition be your guide to sacred sex, but the following ritual may help you better understand just how powerful it can be.

Sacred Sex Ritual

You will need: a bed, candles and holders, condoms (if necessary), and lubricant.

When you and your lover are ready to begin, follow these steps:

1. Arrange the candles in a circle around the room. Make sure your condoms, lubricant, a glass of water, and anything else you might need are nearby.

2. Light the candles and create sacred space.

3. You and your lover should sit on the bed facing each other. Spend time looking at each other. See the divine in your lover.

4. Now "look" at each other with your hands by slowly caressing every inch of each other's bodies. Make sure you maintain eye contact.

5. Replace your fingers with your lips. Move slowly over your lover's body. The goal is not climax, but pleasure. The goal is to build the connection between you, to honor each other's sexual, sensual natures.

6. Come together in the Tantric sitting position. Rock together, letting the pleasure and the spiritual connection intensify as you continue to eye-gaze and couple-breathe.

7. As the moment of climax nears, you will feel spirit fill you. It's almost like being intoxicated or dizzy. Welcome it. Breathe it in.

8. After you've climaxed, lie together on the bed cuddling, kissing, reveling in the physical and spiritual connection you share. Once you've recovered enough to be coherent, share how this experience was different from other times you've made love.

9. Release the sacred space.

Part Two

Enhancing Rituals & Blessings

Although all the rituals and blessings in this book are designed to improve different aspects of your relationship with your lover, the rituals in this section are the foundation for relationship magic. Repeat them as often as you like or need to, and feel free to adapt them to suit the needs of your relationship.

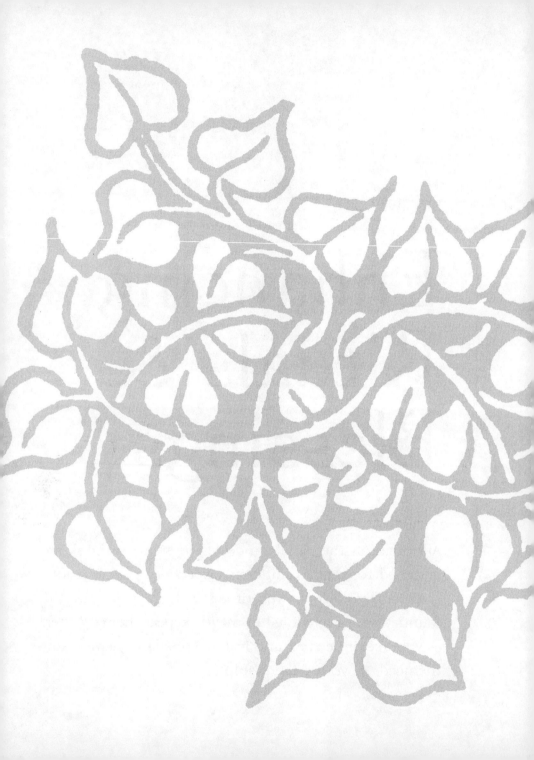

Chapter 11

GRATITUDE RITUAL

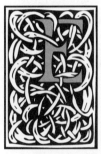very day I see how blessed my life is to have my lover in it. I know he spoils me, and believe me, I am grateful for it. Our friends tease us because of how often we thank each other. Even if we're just sitting on the couch watching television, one of us will look at the other and say, "Thank you. Thank you for being alive and for being who you are. Thank you for loving me. Thank you for letting me love you."

Still, I sometimes forget to tell my lover how grateful I am for him and everything he does for me. I say thank you a million times a day, to everyone from the mail carrier to the checkout clerk at the grocery store, but I don't always remember to thank my lover. Oh sure, I thank him for major things like getting out of bed at 5 A.M. to drive me to the airport, but then I forget to say thank you for lugging my recycling downstairs to the bin.

I devised this gratitude ritual to make sure my lover knows how much I appreciate him. Perform it at your love altar on a night when you can spend the entire evening uninterrupted. Each of you should spend a few days prior to the ritual getting into the "gratitude frame of mind."

The first time my lover and I set out to make our gratitude lists, it was harder than I thought it would be. I wanted mine to be perfect and profound. Then I realized it didn't need to be profound or perfect to be meaningful. It simply needed to be sincere. In fact, I discovered that the small things meant the most.

Once you start thinking about your gratitude lists, include everything that comes to mind, no matter how seemingly insignificant. Don't edit your thoughts, with one caveat: there are no *ifs* or *buts* on this list. It's a gratitude list, not a "to do" list. So don't write, "I thank you for cleaning the tub, but I wish you'd do it more often." Leave it at "I thank you for cleaning the tub," or "I am grateful to you for cleaning the tub."

Gratitude Ritual

You will need: two pieces of parchment paper, two red pens, a pink candle, rose petals, love oil, a night alone with your lover

When you are ready to perform the ritual, follow these steps:

1. Arrange your love altar and gather your supplies.

2. Get into comfortable clothes, if you plan to wear any at all. (It's delicious to perform this ritual naked.)

3. Bring yourselves into sacred space, including your bed in the circle. You'll probably need it.

4. Sitting across from each other, invite Aphrodite to join you:

   "Lady Aphrodite, join us in our rite of gratitude, as we prepare to thank each other for the blessings we bring to the relationship we share. Inspire our hearts and our words with your poetry."

5. Light the candle.

6. Using red pens, write your gratitude lists on the parchment paper.

7. Take turns reading them aloud. Look into each other's eyes as you do this. It may take the rest of the night because if you perform this ritual correctly, you will need to take several kissing, cuddling, and lovemaking breaks. Continue reading your lists after each interlude until you reach the end.

8. Draw the love symbol with love oil at the top of each list, then place them on your love altar. Ask Aphrodite to bless them:

   "Lady Aphrodite, thank you for inspiring our hearts. Please infuse our lists with your blessings, and the energy of love eternal."

9. Couple-breathe and eye-gaze to raise the energy. When the energy is zinging between your heart centers, release it into your lists. Pick them up and say:

   "These lists are charged with love."

10. Release Aphrodite by saying:

    "Thank you for participating in our rite tonight. Stay if you will, go if you must. Farewell and blessed be."

11. Leave the lists on your altar until the next full moon. After they have been charged, you can leave them on your altar, store them in a safe place, or frame them and hang them over your love altar.

12. Whenever you feel doubtful about your relationship, refer to your gratitude lists and see what you can add. They should evolve along with your relationship. You may want to repeat this ritual once a year.

Chapter 12

ROMANCE RITUAL

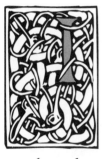love romance. I can't help it. Romance is (and should be) a vital part of every relationship no matter how long you've been together. Most couples know this, yet once the relationship is established they allow themselves to get comfortable and stop working at making it a success. You're too comfortable in your relationship when you stop kissing your lover hello or when you can no longer remember the rush you felt when your eyes first met across a crowded room.

If you've been together a long time, it is more important than ever to keep the romance alive. This can be as simple as sharing a meal at a nice restaurant and *not* talking about your kids, your jobs, your finances, or the lawn that needs mowing, but instead reminiscing about your relationship. Plan an evening-long seduction at least once every month or so.

If it seems that you're always too busy to set aside time for romance, ask yourself why. What is more important than your relationship? In the end, your career, your credit cards, and your over-grown lawn will not matter. Your lover and your children will matter.

At least once a year, and not just on your anniversary, find a way to take that trip you've been yearning for, dine at that fancy restaurant you've been thinking about, and lavish your time and attention only on each other. The surprise of it will heighten the experience.

That said, romance need not be a grand gesture. Sometimes all you need to do is leave a note in your lover's underwear drawer that says, "I love you." Tuck a card into your lover's briefcase or purse. Use your lipstick on the bathroom mirror to tell him how much you'll miss him all day. E-mail your lover a proposition in the the afternoon. Call his voicemail and leave a steamy message. Write a poem. It doesn't have to be a Shakespearean sonnet; the effort alone will be appreciated. All of us, men and women alike, love to receive flowers. Just one is enough, left on the pillow. Frame a photo from a time you both recall as being especially romantic or meaningful. You get the idea. It doesn't matter what you do, as long as you get the message across that you still love your lover as much as you did the first time you said those three little words.

It is also appropriate to turn romance into a ritual. But before you begin, set the stage. Make sure you will be alone for the evening. Don't accept other invitations. Treat the kids to a sleep-over with friends. Turn the ringer off on the phone, and don't even think about turning on the TV. Let your lover know that you will be enjoying each other's company for the whole evening or weekend. Give your lover a little hint of what is to come. The anticipation will fuel you both for the entire day leading up to it.

Create a romantic atmosphere with candles, soft lighting, sumptuous food and drink, and romantic music. Prepare as much of the meal beforehand as you can. A simple, light menu won't weigh you down or take up your time and energy. One of my favorites is cheese fondue served with French bread and good wine. It's filling, but not too filling, and it's fun feed each other. And for dessert, try oranges and strawberries dipped in a chocolate fondue or drizzled with a chocolate wine sauce and served over pound cake. Be sure to lick up any drips—wherever they may fall!

If you need lubricant, condoms, or anything else for lovemaking, be sure they're handy before you start the ritual. You don't want to have to interrupt the proceedings at a crucial moment.

On the evening of the ritual, take a relaxing bath. Quiet your mind so you can focus completely on the romance. Ask your lover to do the same. I wouldn't advise sharing a bath until later in the evening. Once you've bathed, dress in loose-fitting robes, or nothing at all.

Romance Ritual

You will need: good food, fine wine, champagne, or another beverage, lubricant, sensual clothing or lingerie or no clothing, romantic music, candles, a weekend alone together

When you are both ready, begin the ritual.

1. Create sacred space. For this ritual, include your entire home. Banish all everyday thoughts from your mind and focus entirely on the evening at hand.

2. Ask the deity to bring romance to your evening and help you reconnect with each other:

   "O great goddess of love, please add your gift of romance to our night. Help us reconnect. Bring us passion, love, and joy."

3. Next, it is time for dinner. Remember to feed each other and find creative and sensual ways to take care of spills.

4. During dessert, take the time to communicate with each other, but not about work, or school, or bills. Talk about each other. Talk about how much you love and appreciate your life together. Reminisce about when you met. Remind each other why you were first attracted to one another. Share your fantasies.

5. As you become more emotionally intimate, it's time to move the scene to lovemaking. Slow and passionate is the rule. Instead of rushing to intercourse, tease each other. You have all night. Visit each other's pleasure spots, and then try to find new ones.

6. The love doesn't have to end after lovemaking. After you've renewed your physical and emotional connections, spend time cuddling in each other's arms, stroking each other's skin, and gazing into each other's eyes. Enjoy the feeling of your lover's body entwined with yours. Revel in the experience of the two of you wrapped in your personal cocoon. If sleep calls you, go with it. If your lover awakens you in the middle of the night for a little nocturnal nuzzling, why not?

7. The next morning, make breakfast together, wearing whatever you feel comfortable in. For my lover and I, that is often nothing. (Watch for splatters!) Be lazy together. Sit on the couch and read the newspaper wrapped in each other's

arms until the mood to make love strikes you again and let that happen wherever you are. This is your day to forget about the world and become completely absorbed in each other as you celebrate your relationship.

8. When you must finally bring your time together to an end, thank the goddess for blessing your evening:

"O great goddess of love, thank you for giving us the gift of romance. Please extend your blessing for all our days together. Stay if you will, go if you must. Farewell and blessed be."

9. Release your sacred space.

10. Place a rose petal on your nightstand or love altar as a constant reminder of this time you spent together.

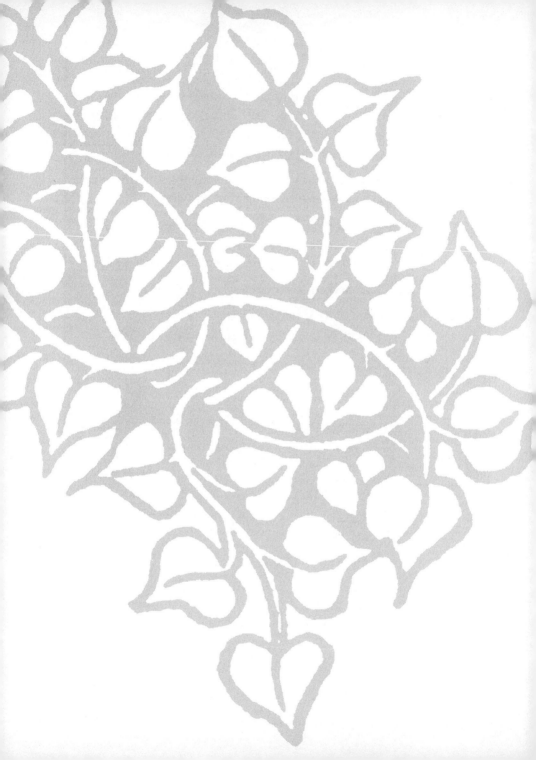

Chapter 13

THE GREAT RITE

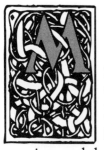y lover and I are part of a Wiccan circle. Every May we celebrate the ancient Celtic fertility festival called Beltane, also known as May Day. Beltane is a wonderfully sexy day filled with bawdy energy and high passion, and the perfect opportunity to practice the Great Rite. This ritual symbolizes the union of the god and goddess as they consummate their courtship. You can recreate their union any day or night of the year, but Beltane Eve is the traditional time to do it.

First, if you can find a local maypole, by all means join in the festivities. As you probably know, in many cultures and countries the maypole is a phallic symbol around which a fertility rite is performed. Although the fertility aspect of the maypole dance is not restricted to human reproduction, but also refers to creativity in general, engaging in the dance is a great way to get your heart pumping, and your passion raging. Once you return home, you'll scarcely be able to keep your hands off each other.

Be aware, the energy of Beltane is very potent. If you and your lover don't want to become pregnant, use the appropriate precautions when performing the Great Rite.

Before you begin this ritual, have everything handy, including lubricant, condoms, and crowns. Use flower crowns, leaf crowns, newspaper crowns, or even Burger King crowns. It really doesn't matter. Have fun. As the newly crowned King and Queen of the May, your duty is to have madly passionate sex. Lose yourselves in it. If you have something special you'd like to ask for that affects you as a couple, such as conceiving a child, then use the energy of your May Day lovemaking to acquire it. Keep it in your consciousness as the goal of your lovemaking. Sexual energy has amazing power. Of course, you needn't have a goal beyond having great sex, which in and of itself will have a fabulous effect on your relationship.

After you have finished the Great Rite, and it may take hours, revel in the afterglow by reaffirming your love for and commitment to each other. Use May Day to celebrate being together. Champagne or sparkling cider in bed is the perfect thirst-quencher after all the erotic adventures of the day.

As a final touch, keep your crowns in the bedroom until the following year. Ours are hanging from the bedposts as a reminder of the wonderful Great Rite we shared on Beltane.

The Great Rite

You will need: crowns, candles, lubricant, condoms (if needed), a romantic setting

When you are ready to begin the ritual, follow these steps:

1. Create sacred space.

2. Invite the goddess and god to join you.

   "Aphrodite, watcher of lovers, goddess of passion, lying in the moonlight, uniting us in love, come join us in our celebration this Beltane evening. Eros, protector of mates, god of sensuality, running under the sun, uniting us in love, come join us in our celebration this Beltane evening."

3. As you sit facing each other, place the crown on the Queen's head, saying:

   "I crown you Queen of the May, embodiment of all that is sensual and exciting."

4. As you place the crown on the King's head, say:

   "I crown you King of the May, embodiment of all that is sexual and passionate."

5. Move into the Tantric sitting position and begin kissing, caressing, and moving toward lovemaking. Go slowly, covering every inch of each other's bodies.

6. Couple-breathe and eye-gaze as much as possible to heighten the energy between you.

7. When you must release, do so.

8. After you have both reached orgasm, lie in each other's arms to recover from the outpouring of energy.

9. Release the goddess and god.

"We thank you Aphrodite, watcher of mates, goddess of sensuality, for watching over us this Beltane eve. We thank you Eros, protector of lovers, god of passion, for watching over us this Beltane eve."

10. Release your sacred space.

Chapter 14

REKINDLING LOVE

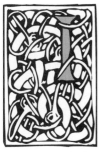f the flame of love is threatening to wink out, and dating isn't doing the trick, add a morning cuddle or prayer to your daily routine. If you choose a prayer, you can say it together. My lover and I prefer a morning cuddle, but I add a request to my daily prayer and meditation later. I ask that my connection with my lover stays strong and clear, that our passion doesn't fade, and that we don't lose the love from our lives.

I pray and meditate after I get up, so the cuddle comes before I get out bed. I am the last person willing to give up sleep time, but waking up five minutes early for some close-togetherness time before the day begins is worth it, believe me. It is so wonderful to curl up under the warm covers with my lover and just be with him for a few minutes.

You probably did this at the beginning of your relationship. If you've stopped, it's time to re-establish this intimate time. Tell each other how happy you are to be together, share your gratitude, express your feelings—but no complaining. Keep the complaints out of your bed!

Looking after your altar is another way to keep love kindled. Make sure it's neat and current. Replace the flower before it dies, and wash the altar cloth if it gets dusty or stained. Make tending your altar, and your love, a joint project. If you've let your altar go a little bit, perform this brief ritual for relighting the flame and recharging the energy.

Recharging Your Love Altar

You will need: love oil, a pink candle, a clean altar cloth, a broom

When you have everything gathered, follow these steps:

1. Give the room a psychic cleaning with your broom, just as you did when you first built your altar.

2. Cast the circle around your entire bedroom or wherever your altar is located. Call the quarters and elements to join you.

3. Invite Aphrodite, or another goddess if you prefer, to attend your ritual.

   "Lady Aphrodite, goddess of love, passion, and romance, please join us as we recharge our altar to enhance our love. Bless it with your powers of love, that it may keep the flame of our love burning for all time."

4. When you need to wash or replace your altar cloth, carefully remove everything before you arrange the clean or new

cloth. You can re-bless your altar objects if you like, but it's not necessary. You may wish to replace some of the items, in which case you do need to bless those.

5. Is your pink candle burned out? Filled with dust? If it's still usable, you can keep it, otherwise replace it. Either way, put a new coat of oil on its surface, drawing the oil from the top and bottom edges into the middle. As you do this, visualize drawing love to yourselves.

6. Set the pink candle in its holder in the middle of the altar. Light it now and say:

"We relight the flame to recharge our love. The passion of fire and the warmth of love have returned to our lives."

7. The crystal may also need to be cleansed and recharged. To cleanse it, set it on rock salt for three days. When you place the crystal back on the altar, recharge it by saying:

"This crystal is the physical manifestation of our love. May it amplify our feelings and encourage happiness."

8. When your altar is clean, items replaced or updated, and your candle burning, join hands, eye-gaze, and couple-breathe. As you breathe together, feel the energy around you expanding to the altar. Focus on infusing the altar with love. When you feel the energy has reached a high point, turn to the altar and say:

"This altar is a testament to our love. It is blessed with the powers of love that it may keep the flame of our love burning for all time. So mote it be."

Release all the energy into the altar.

9. Thank Aphrodite for her blessing and say:

"Lady Aphrodite, goddess of love, passion, and romance, thank you for joining us as we recharge our altar to enhance our love. Thank you for blessing it with your powers of love that it may keep the flame of our love burning for all time."

10. Release your sacred space.

11. Feel free to make love to seal the altar blessing.

Chapter 15

RESTORING PASSION

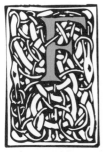or some, passion is like two trees in a forest fire, but for others it is more like a self-renewing candle that never burns out, slow, steady, and always there. Sometimes, the passion goes out completely. Maybe you've both been working late or spending hours arguing the kids into bed every night. Maybe there is a medical or physical reason for the problem. Whatever it is, all you want to do at night is collapse on the couch in front of the television. Romance and sex are the last things on your mind. That's no good! No relationship will last if you don't give it a little nourishment and encouragement.

Like all couples, my lover and I had periods when the passion wasn't running high for any number of reasons. But we've never been willing to just accept the situation. We've always made an effort to bring passion back into our relationship. The ritual below is one method we have used to get things sizzling again.

Every time my lover and I perform this ritual, I am overwhelmed with love for him. I languish in the sensation of touching him and am loathe to separate from him. I hope it works this way for you.

When you decide it's time to do the ritual, make sure the kids are asleep, and turn off the television, telephone, cell phone, fax machine, computer, and pager. No one needs to reach you that badly. Now, go into the bedroom and lock the door. Remember the sacred sex I mentioned earlier? You are about to experience it.

Restoring Passion Ritual

What you will need: a red candle, love oil, red sheets, lubricant, rose petals

When you have everything, begin the ritual.

1. Come into sacred space, however you choose to do this.

2. Light the red candle and ask Aphrodite and Eros to join you and say:

   "Aphrodite, goddess of sensuality, Eros, god of sexuality, please join us as we restore our passion. Bless us with your gifts of desire and arousal."

3. Now, don't go rushing into sex. I want you to cherish each other. Sit cross-legged facing each other and hold hands. Spend a few minutes eye-gazing and couple-breathing. Feel the connection this creates between you.

4. Reach out and lovingly stroke each other's faces. Revel in the sensation of caressing and being caressed.

5. When you are ready, slowly remove one item of your lover's clothing. Cherish the skin underneath. Anoint it with love oil. Kiss it tenderly. Smell it. Touch it. Feel it. Remember it. Trace your fingertips ever so gently over the exposed skin. Your lover should do the same for you.

6. Remove each piece of clothing until you are both naked. You will both be extremely aroused by now, but it's not time for intercourse yet. Come into the Tantric sitting position and continue eye-gazing, couple-breathing, kissing, and caress-ing. Make as much contact with your bodies as you can. Love every inch of your lover's skin.

7. Rock your bodies together. Feel how excited you become when your genitals touch. Feel the connection between them. Only when you feel that further delaying intercourse will surely kill you, should you come together in the most intimate union.

8. Rock slowly together. Try not to begin rapid thrusting. Instead, slowly work up the pace. Keep your eyes trained on each other. Bring your breathing into unison again. Really feel your connection.

9. I promise you, you will both reach amazing climaxes, but delay them as long as possible. You may want to take breaks to just sit together, without separating, and kiss. Not moving. Just feeling.

10. Once you have climaxed, remain in the Tantric sitting position while you recover.

11. In the morning, release Aphrodite and Eros and say:

"Aphrodite, goddess of sensuality, Eros, god of sexuality, thank you for joining us as we restored the passion. We are honored by your gifts."

12. Release your sacred space.

Couples with physical challenges to intercourse can still perform this ritual. Lengthen the time you spend caressing and cuddling, shift into positions that allow each of you to give and receive pleasure. Regardless of whether or not you both climax, make sure that you both feel cherished, loved, and pleasured.

Chapter 16

CREATING FIREWORKS

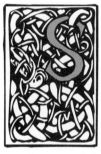

Sometimes a couple needs a little jump-start as opposed to major engine work, as in the restoring passion ritual. Or maybe you've done the restoring passion ritual and want to give it a little boost when you're both in the mood, but just can't get up the energy for a sexy romp.

This happens to me on occasion. I have so much to do, that sometimes I'm just too tired and distracted and even though I want to make love, I just can't get into the right mood, which frustrates my lover. I find that a little jump-starter is exactly what I need to get things going again.

In this ritual, you will bless a candle to spark your sensual fireworks. Once you've created the candle, burn it for at least fifteen minutes each time you need a sexual boost.

Candle Blessing

What you will need: a red candle, gold glitter, love oil

When you are ready to begin, use the following ritual.

1. Create sacred space.

2. Invite Aphrodite and Eros to join you by saying:

   "Lady and lord of passion, Aphrodite and Eros, we call you. Please join us as we create a fresh spark to ignite our relationship fireworks."

3. Hold the candle between you as you eye-gaze and couple-breathe to raise energy. Your intention is to charge the candle with passion so it will create fireworks each time you light it.

4. Dress the candle in love oil by drawing the oil from the bottom up to the middle and from the top down to the middle, thereby drawing in love.

5. Roll the candle in glitter.

6. Set the candle in the holder and say:

   "This candle is blessed. May it set off our internal fireworks each time it is lit."

7. Light the candle and make passionate love.

8. Release Aphrodite and Eros. Say:

   "Lady and lord of passion, Aphrodite and Eros, we thank you for joining us as we created a fresh spark of passion and love. We are blessed and honored by your presence. Stay if you will, go if you must. Farewell and blessed be."

9. Release your sacred space.

10. When your relationship starts to feel flat, light the candle and let the fireworks explode.

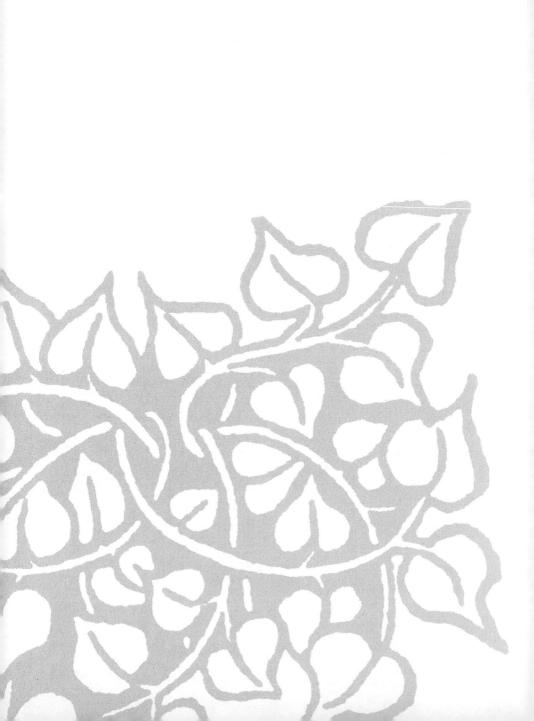

Chapter 17

ENSURING A LASTING RELATIONSHIP

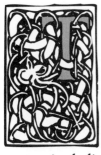he goal of this book is to give you some tools to help keep your relationship strong and enduring. Remind yourselves why you chose one another in the first place; revisit your marriage vows and review your gratitude lists once a year. Rewrite them, and in a special ritual, burn the old ones and empower the new. Or place your old gratitude lists in a special box to preserve them so that you can look back on how your values and relationship have evolved.

Use the rituals in this book to help you work through the difficult times, but also to honor the good ones. Honor the differences between you and respect your separate interests. Perhaps in addition to your gratitude lists, create honoring lists. List everything you appreciate and admire about your lover's personality. These are not necessarily things that your lover does for you, or

🍂 65

should do for you. They are things that are special to or unique about your lover. For example:

I honor your web design skills.

I honor your ability to let go of a grievance.

I honor your ability to forgive.

I honor your silly smile.

I honor your desire to keep that 15-year-old shirt.

Using the ritual below, read your new gratitude and honoring lists to each other. You may wish you could participate more in your lover's outside interests, but be careful. If you are genuinely interested in learning about or joining in them, then by all means do so. But if you are only doing so because you think you *should* want to share in everything your lover does, then hold off. It is important to have your own interests, your own personality, your own hobbies, and your own friends.

Blessing a Lasting Relationship

What you will need: a pink candle, love oil, parchment paper, red pens

When you are ready to begin, follow these steps:

1. Come into sacred space.

2. Invite Aphrodite to join you with words such as:

"Lady Aphrodite, join us as we prepare to honor each other for our own unique blessings and the unique blessings we bring to the relationship we share. Inspire our hearts and our words with your poetry."

3. Light the pink candle.

4. Using red pens, write your lists on parchment paper.

5. After you've finished, take turns reading the individual items aloud until you've each read through your lists. Look into each other's eyes as you do this.

6. Draw the love symbol with love oil at the top of each list, then place the lists on your love altar. Ask Aphrodite to bless them with words such as:

"Lady Aphrodite, thank you for inspiring our hearts. Please infuse our lists with your blessings, and the energy of love eternal."

7. Couple-breathe and eye-gaze to raise the energy. When the energy is zinging between your heart centers, release it into your lists. Pick them up and say:

"These lists are charged with love."

8. Release Aphrodite with words such as:

"Thank you for participating in our rite tonight. Stay if you will, go if you must. Farewell and blessed be."

Leave the lists on your altar until the next full moon.

9. After the lists have been charged, put them in a safe place. As with the gratitude lists, they should evolve along with your relationship.

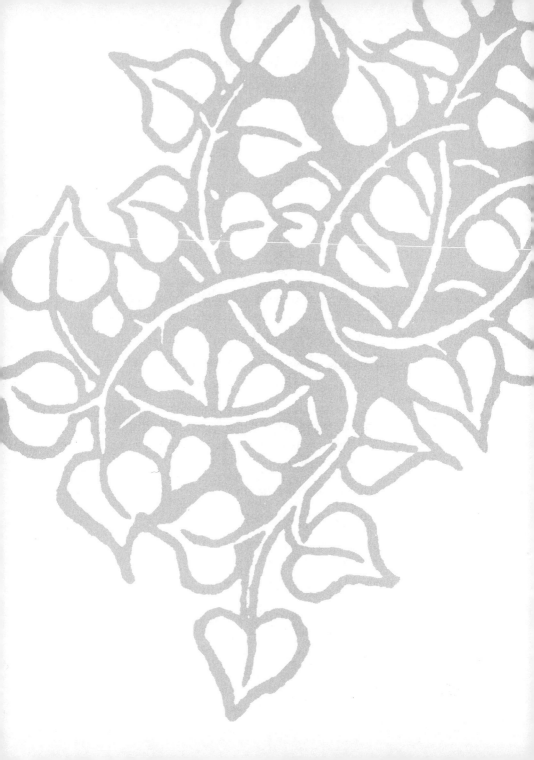

Chapter 18

FUN TIME RITUAL

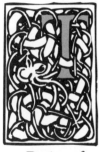his is actually not a ritual. Sometimes we just need to get away, for no other reason than to relax and have fun. It's not about romance. It's not about communication. It's about fun. It's about continuing to date. Dating after you've been together a long time? You betcha.

My lover and I have been together a long time, but we still go hiking, go to the movies, and play miniature golf, and we still call them dates. We still make the plans in advance, when possible. We still say, "Do you want to do something on Saturday?" This makes it feel more like a date.

So, this ritual is really just a date. This means that you make your plans ahead of time, just like for a date. One of you has to pick the other up, just like on a date. Sex is not guaranteed at the end of the night. Well, okay, you can skip that rule. But try to get some anticipation in there. If you're going to the movies, choose something exciting that will get your adrenaline going. Horror and action movies are aphrodisiacs. If you're going miniature golfing or participating in some other competitive activity, make it into a contest, with an erotic prize going to the winner. Dinner and dancing are also excellent choices. Make sure you work up a good sweat on the dance floor and keep your heart racing all the way home.

Where's the ritual in all this? There isn't really, and that's exactly the point. No creating sacred space, no invoking a deity. Before you leave on your date, promise each other that you will have fun—just the two of you. Leave your pagers, cell phones, and Palm Pilots at home. Then go out and just do it.

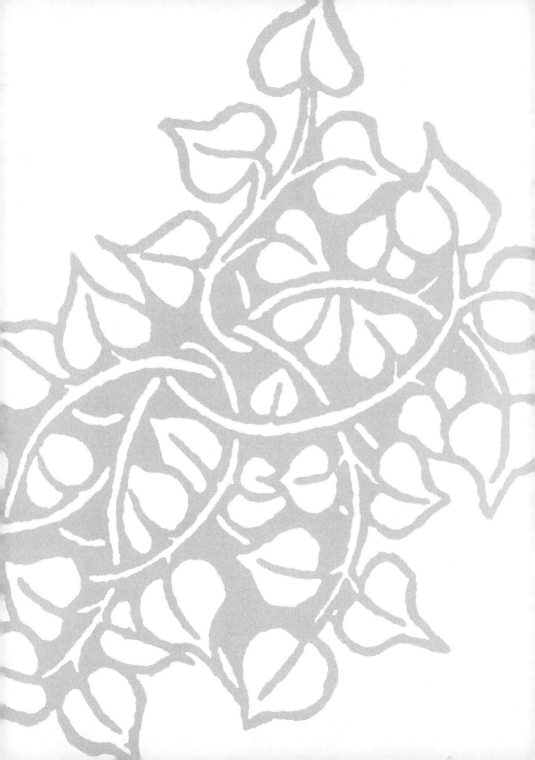

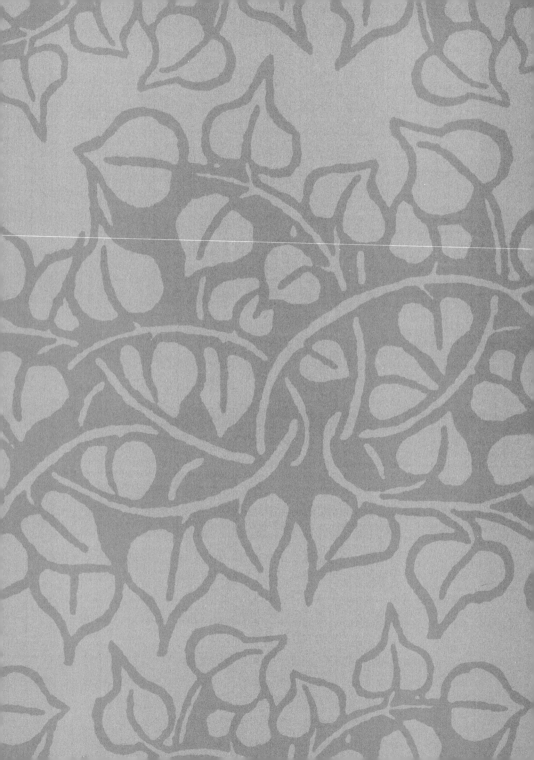

Part Three

Uniting Ceremonies & Blessings

Uniting ceremonies and blessings are designed to join you and your lover together in a more committed relationship. If you're already legally married, you may still wish to have a uniting ceremony. If you don't wish to be legally married, but do want to formally state your commitment to each other, there is a ritual for this also. Families may also be ceremonially united.

Certain relationship milestones can strengthen or weaken your bond: the first time you meet each other's parents or your first holiday together, for instance. Your uniting ceremony may be a one-time-only occasion or something you do every year or every ten years. Do whatever feels right for you, your relationship, and your family.

Chapter 19

MEET THE PARENTS

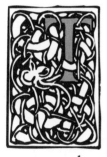he first time you meet your lover's parents can be stressful, especially if you plan on spending the rest of your life with your lover. Even the most well-intentioned parents will make judgments about you and appraise your worthiness for their child. Don't take it personally. It is their parental duty to look out for their child's best interests.

If you and your lover are anxious about this first meeting, consider using this ritual to help you get through it.

Meet the Parents Ceremony

What you will need: love altar, a photo of you and your lover

When you are ready to begin, follow these steps:

1. Create sacred space around your love altar.

2. Ask the goddess Hestia to join you by saying:

"Lady Hestia, goddess of hearth and home, please bless us as we bless ourselves before (name) meets (name)'s parents. Please help to make this introduction peaceful, warm, and comfortable."

3. Join hands and look into each other's eyes.

The lover whose parents are being met says:

"I promise not to become so involved in my family that I forget to pay attention to you."

The lover who is meeting the parents says:

"I promise to be friendly and not withdraw when anxious or nervous."

4. Together, say:

"We promise not to make any embarrassing comments."

5. Eye-gaze and couple-breathe to raise energy. When you feel the energy has reached a high point, the lover whose parents are being met says:

"Lady Hestia, please help my parents to be accepting and warm toward (name). I ask this for the good of all. And it harm none, so mote it be."

6. Thank and release Hestia:

"Lady Hestia, goddess of hearth and home, thank you for guaranteeing this meeting will be smooth and joyous. Thank you for joining in our rite. Stay if you will, go if you must. Farewell and blessed be."

7. Release your sacred space.

Chapter 20

FIRST HOLIDAY TOGETHER

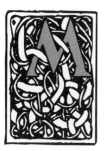y lover and I spent our first Yule together only two months after we had started dating. It was a busy month, but we still found time to be alone together. One of those times was the night we decorated my tree. While we didn't follow the ritual that follows exactly, it was so helpful for us. You might find it helpful in alleviating some of the relationship stress that might otherwise ruin your first major holiday together.

Before you begin, find or make a special ornament to go on the tree. The ornament will be a surprise for your lover.

You can adapt this ritual to any holiday. For example, if your first major holiday is Valentine's Day, instead of an ornament, make or decorate a special frame for a photo that you will take on this day.

Blessing Your First Holiday Together

You will need: Yule tree or other holiday symbol, a special holiday ornament, champagne or wine or eggnog. If this ritual is done at Yule, it should be performed after you have put up your tree and strung the lights.

When you are ready to begin, follow these steps:

1. Create sacred space around your tree.

2. Invite the goddess to join you by saying:

   "Great goddess, please join us as we celebrate our first holiday together. May it be the first of many."

3. Decorate your tree with all of your ornaments except the secret one.

4. When the tree is fully decorated, produce the gift for your lover.

5. After your lover has opened the gift, sit facing each other, holding the ornament together. Bless the ornament by saying:

   "This ornament is a symbol of our relationship. It is but the first of many that will fill our lives. May it serve as a reminder of this special day."

6. Couple-breathe and eye-gaze to raise energy and bless the ornament. When the energy is full, direct it into the ornament and say:

   "This ornament is blessed."

7. Have your lover place the ornament on a central branch of the tree.

8. Kiss, hug, make love if you feel so moved, to emphasize the blessing.

9. Release the goddess, saying:

   "Great goddess, thank you for joining us as we celebrate our first holiday together. It is but the first of many. Thank you for your blessings. Stay if you will, go it you must. Farewell and blessed be."

10. Release your sacred space.

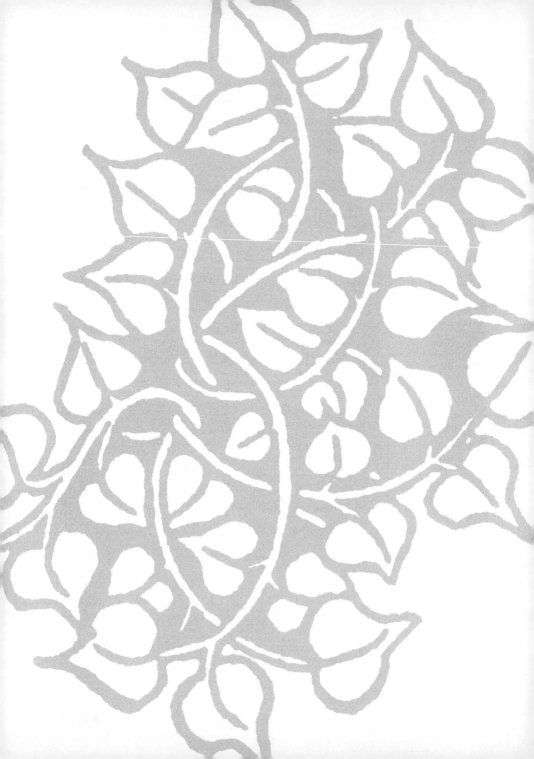

Chapter 21

PRIVATE HANDFASTING

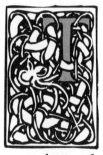here may come a time when you and your lover wish
to have a commitment ceremony rather than a legally
binding marriage. Use the public handfasting ritual,
if you want to include your family and friends and
make it a formal event. If you prefer it to be just the two of you,
then perform a private handfasting ceremony. Married couples
wishing to renew their vows but without a formal ceremony may
also perform this ritual.

First, choose a private place. A natural setting is ideal—near
a waterfall, in a meadow, in the woods, on a beach—you get the
idea. If you can afford it, you might take a vacation to a romantic
spot and hold the ceremony there. If you're in a place that would
make an outdoor ceremony uncomfortable or impractical, such as
Michigan in January, create a romantic setting in your home with
candlelight, beautiful music, and an elegant meal.

A day or two before the ceremony, you will need to braid three silk cords together or make a flower chain. You will also need rings or you can make wreaths for your heads out of flowers, vines, or lacy fabric. If flowers and greenery are abundant, and you are skilled at making handicrafts, you can fashion your cords and crowns on the spot.

Once everything is in place, you should each take a moment to think about what this ceremony means and be sure it is really what you want. Write down your vows if you plan to say something formal. If you are a confidant public speaker, wait until the right moment and see what comes to you. A wonderful option is to incorporate sentiments from your gratitude lists as promises that you intend to keep within your relationship.

Private Handfasting Ceremony

What you will need: silk cord, two crowns or wreaths or rings, a romantic setting, written vows

When the time for your uniting ceremony has arrived, follow these steps:

1. Go to the location you have chosen with all your supplies.

2. When you are ready, sit down cross-legged facing each other. Join hands. Say together:

   "God and goddess of love, please join us as we unite ourselves in love. We do this in honor of you and to honor each other and our relationship. Lend us your blessings on this special day."

3. Now, pick up one crown and place it on your lover's head, or slip a ring on your lover's finger, then join hands again. Looking into your lover's eyes, state your vows in your own words. An example would be:

"I promise before all the universe to love and respect you for as long as the elements shall blow with the wind, flow with the water, burn with the flame, and support us on this earth."

4. Your lover repeats the procedure for you and speaks his or her vows. Another example might be:

"I swear before all the powers that be, this waterfall, the sun overhead, the wind in the trees, and the earth beneath my feet, that my love for you will grow as we grow together."

5. Cross your wrists and join hands with your lover. Wrap the cord twice around your lover's wrists to make a loop. Now wrap it loosely around your own wrist. You may need to remove your other hand to tie the ends of the cord together, being careful to maintain your "empty" loop. Then slide both of your hands back into the loop, cross your wrists, and rejoin hands with your lover. Together say:

"We are bound to each other for as long as our love shall last."

6. Kiss to seal your vows, then slip your hands out of the cord, but leave it tied. The tied cord will serve as a symbol of your promises.

7. Thank and release the god and goddess by saying:

"God and goddess of love, thank you for witnessing our union and for blessing us on this special day. Stay if you will, go if you must. Farewell and blessed be."

8. Release your sacred space.

9. Stay and celebrate with food and drink, or go home to celebrate there. If you wore crowns or wreaths, keep them. Put both the cord and wreaths somewhere you will remember them. Take them out whenever you need to be reminded of your commitment. You can also display them somewhere in your home. If you chose to exchange rings, wear them as you would wedding or engagement rings.

10. Just as you would on your wedding night, make love to consummate your union.

Chapter 22

PUBLIC HANDFASTING

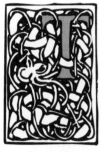his ceremony can be performed in place of a traditional wedding. It is legally binding if your officiant is licensed by your state. It is also an appropriate ceremony if you and your lover are gay and wish to be formally united. Included here is a sample ritual that can be adapted or altered to suit your needs.

As with all weddings, legal or symbolic, this one will require planning ahead. In fact, a traditional wedding planning book may provide helpful advice. In addition to rings, you will need a cord for this ceremony. Make a braid from cords of three different colors. Choose colors that represent the properties you wish to bring to your marriage. Examples include: red for love, green for prosperity, blue for good health and communication, yellow for joy, and purple for spiritual growth. (See Appendix C for more on colors and their meanings.) Research and choose colors that have special meaning for you.

This ceremony also includes the ritual of cakes and ale. You can use small pieces of your wedding cake, or a small cake baked especially for this purpose. Mead, wine, champagne, or juice, depending on your preference, may be substituted for the ale.

The clothing you wear, again, depends on your preference: a theme-appropriate costume, a flowing white gown and bare feet, or a tasteful dress or suit are all options.

Some couples like to provide printed explanations of the various elements used in the ceremony for their guests. As examples, the braided cord is a traditional Celtic symbol that is still sometimes used in Ireland today. The cakes and ale are an offering of sustenance and abundance. The broom is a multicultural symbol of fertility.

If you feel that casting the circle and calling the quarters will confuse some of your guests, you may omit this part of the ritual, or perform them silently or before your guests arrive. Simply cut a "door" in the air where the entrance to the circle will be, then discreetly "close" it when you begin the ceremony.

Finally, you'll need your vows and blessings scrolls. You may select formal vows from a book or write your own. I do recommend writing them ahead of time rather than improvising on the spot. You'll want to remember them after the ceremony, and a spontaneous speech after a long day of celebration may not be so easy to recall.

Your guests will participate by reading a blessing at the end of the ceremony. Have the blessing printed on cards or scrolls and distributed to your guests before the ceremony begins. They will be lovely mementos of your handfasting.

Public Handfasting Ceremony

You will need: silk cord, rings, written vows, someone to officiate, cake, ale, a chalice, a plate, a broom, blessing scrolls

On the day of the wedding, follow these steps:

1. Mark your marriage sacred space by walking in a circle around the altar and area where your guests are seated.

2. The person who is officiating walks to the altar and stands facing your guests, then says:

   "Welcome all who have come today to witness the union of (your names) as they formally promise themselves to each other and, through their handfasting, join their lives together as one. Please stand now as (your names) join us in this celebration of their love."

3. The guests stand and turn to face you as you and your lover walk down the center aisle together. Stand hand-in-hand facing the altar as the officiant invites the elements or other spirits to join you. Use the words from the circle cast or other words you prefer.

4. The officiant invites the goddess to attend the ceremony, saying:

   "O great lady, from whom all love is derived and for whom is known the greatest love, please join this couple today on the occasion of their handfasting. Grant them the blessings of your wisdom as they prepare to spend the remainder of their days together."

   After a moment of silence, the officiant invites the god to join the ceremony, saying:

"O great lord, you who are derived from the goddess's love and desire, please join us today as we bless the union of this couple before you. Grant them the blessings of your passion as they prepare to spend the remainder of their days together."

5. You can ask two of your friends to read the "Charges of the God and Goddess" or read them yourselves. Other prayers may be substituted.

6. When all prayers have been read, the officiant asks you:

   "Do you both come here today of your own free will to be joined before the gods and all who are present here?"

   "Yes," or *"We do,"* is the appropriate answer.

7. The officiant asks,

   "Do you (name) take (name) as your (spouse title)?"

   "I do," or *"Yes,"* is the appropriate answer.

   The officiant repeats for the other lover. Now read your personal vows.

8. The officiant holds up the rings, saying:

   "These rings symbolize the circle of life and the circle of love. By wearing them, (your names) recognize that love and life have their ups and downs, but they always return to the beginning."

9. The officiant places one ring in the hand of the female lover (or whomever you decide will go first) and says:

   "(Name), place this ring on (name)'s finger as a symbol of your dedication to him." Repeat with the other lover.

10. The officiant holds up a plate with two small morsels of cake and a cup of ale, mead, or wine and says:

"(Your names) will now bless each other with sustenance and prosperity through the ceremony of cakes and ale."

Offer the cake to each other with the words:

"May you never hunger."

Repeat with the ale and the words:

"May you never thirst."

11. Join hands with your lover, crossing your wrists. The officiant wraps the cord around your wrists three times, knots the cord, and says:

    "You are bound to each other for as long as your love shall last." (Or *". . . until death parts you."* if you prefer.)

12. Seal your union with a kiss, then slip your hands out of the cord, leaving the knot tied as a symbol of your promises to each other and marriage bond between you.

13. A friend or the officiant should lay a broom on the floor or ground a few steps behind you. With hands joined, turn to face your guests and step over the broom to guarantee prosperity and fertility. Continue facing your guests as the officiant says:

    "These two stand before you today joined as one. They now ask for your blessing."

14. Your guests will now stand and read in unison from their scrolls:

    "(Your names), we served today as witnesses to your blessed union. Now we offer you this wish: May you be healthy, wealthy, and joyous for all the days of your lives."

15. The guests resume their seats and the officiant says:

    "I declare before the gods that you are joined in a sacred union as husband and wife. The ceremony is concluded."

16. The officiant should thank the gods and quarters for their attendance and bid them farewell, then release the circle.

17. It's party time! Enjoy your reception.

Chapter 23

MERGING TWO FAMILIES

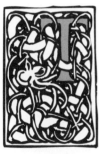 oday, many lovers are coming together with children from previous relationships. To symbolize and solidify the union of this new family, consider including the children in your handfasting ceremony or perform an additional family handfasting ceremony later.

If you are including the children in your public handfasting, ask them to join you at the altar after you and your lover have said your vows. Promise that you will always make time for your children and that your love for them will not diminish in any way. Then, promise the children you will be step-parenting that you will respect and honor them and not attempt to take the place of their other parent. Each child should also vow to respect the two of you, as well as to respect their siblings.

If you are performing your ceremony at home, you can make it more personal. Plan your handfasting as a coming together of the whole family. Do this by holding hands and making a promise to each person in the new family.

Everyone in the household should receive some sort of symbol to remind them that they are now members of a new family, a reminder of the promises that now bind them together. Perhaps give each child a small ring, necklace, or pin they can wear. As an alternative, devise a family symbol and place a copy of it in each bedroom as well as the family room, kitchen, or entryway.

If this is part of your larger handfasting ritual, include your children in the cakes and ale portion, then have them witness your handfasting with the cord. If this is a private handfasting, then adjourn for a family meal that is prepared and eaten together. Continue the celebration with a night of music, dancing, games, or a family outing.

It might also be a good idea to renew your promises once a year, perhaps on the anniversary of your handfasting, to mark the evolution of your new family.

Adapt the framework that follows to suit your family, their cultural backgrounds, ages, and emotional needs.

Merging Two Families Ceremony

You will need: written family vows, family rings or other symbolic items

When you are ready to begin:

1. Create sacred space together. For young children, you may need to explain it as special time.

2. Invite Hera, Demeter, Brighid, or Hestia to join you by saying:

   "Hera, goddess of marriage and family, please join us as we unite our family in mutual love, respect, and affection."

3. Go around the table or altar making your promises to each other.

4. Hold up the rings or family symbol you have chosen. Ask for Hera's blessing:

   "Goddess Hera, this (object) is a symbol of our family union. Please bless it for peace, joy, and honor."

5. Adorn each family member with the symbol.

6. Allow the children to make any final comments.

7. Thank the goddess you have chosen for her blessing by saying:

   "Hera, goddess of marriage and family, thank you for blessing our family and for the blessings of peace, affection, respect, and joy. Stay if you will, go if you must. Farewell and blessed be."

8. Release your sacred space and adjourn to the family meal.

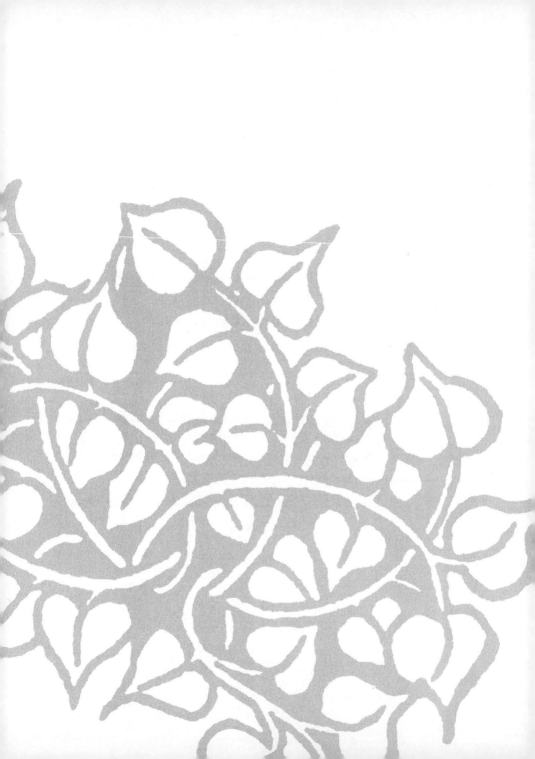

Chapter 24

POST-WEDDING VOWS

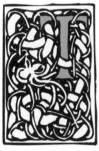he wedding is over. After months of planning and a long day of feasting, dancing, and celebrating with your guests and with each other, you're both exhausted. This ritual can be performed on the first, or any night of your honeymoon, or on your first night at home together after the ceremony. If you have not lived together before your wedding, perform it on the night you move into your new home together. In this case, be sure to have your love altar in place. There is no expiration date for making personal vows. Even if you've been married a long time, you can make your vows tonight.

To make new or post-wedding vows, go back and revisit your gratitude lists. Consider turning some of the things your lover is already grateful for into promises. For example, if your lover appreciates being surprised with breakfast in bed, make a promise to do it more often. Be creative, be specific, and make your vows personally meaningful.

The important thing about post-wedding vows is that you keep them just as you do your wedding vows. If you promise to do something, then do it.

If you start to slip on your promises, review and renew them. Reread them to one another from time to time. And if you call on the goddess Hera for this ritual, be sure to keep those promises. Hera is a powerful protector of marriage and will kick your butt if you fail to keep your vows.

Post-wedding Vows Ceremony

You will need: gratitude lists or vows, love altar, parchment paper, red pens

When you have gathered all your supplies, begin the ritual:

1. Create sacred space together.

2. Invite Hera, Demeter, Brighid, or Hestia to join you by saying:

   "Hera, goddess of marriage, please join us as we make new promises to each other. Please bless us with the gift of a strong union."

3. Write your vows now on the parchment and then read them aloud.

4. Place your vows on the altar and draw the love symbol on the parchment paper with love oil.

5. Join hands, eye-gaze, and couple-breathe to raise energy. Feel your heart centers connect, then expand the energy to encompass your love altar and vows you've made. Feel your vows energizing your relationship.

6. When the energy is full, together say:

   "I promise to keep my vows to you, to the best of my ability and for all time. May I never forget to love, honor, and cherish you and our love."

7. Thank Hera for joining you:

   "Goddess Hera, protector of marriage, the promises we have made, please help us keep them. Thank you for your blessings. Stay if you will, go if you must. Farewell and blessed be."

8. Release your sacred space unless you wish to make love to add an extra blessing to your vows.

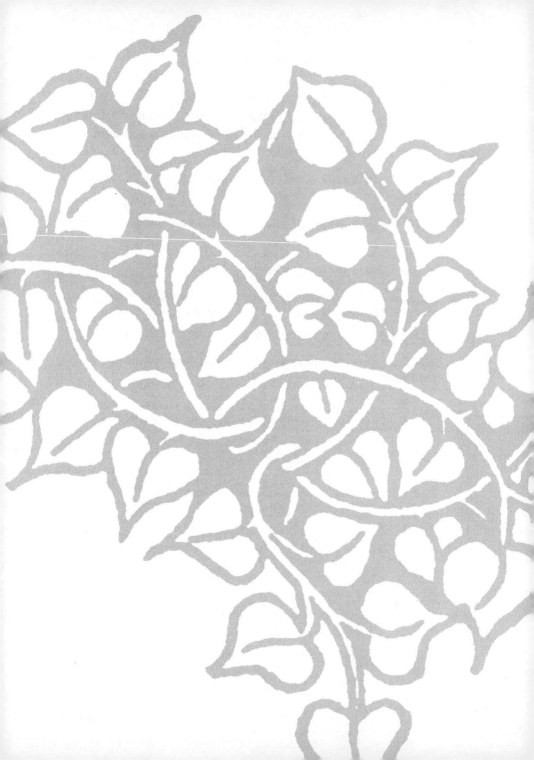

Chapter 25

PREPARING FOR A CHILD

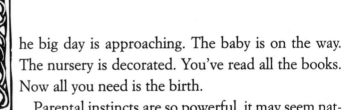he big day is approaching. The baby is on the way. The nursery is decorated. You've read all the books. Now all you need is the birth.

Parental instincts are so powerful, it may seem natural to allow your relationship with your lover to come second to the new child. Of course, children have overwhelming needs. Their health, happiness, and safety are in your hands. But if you and your lover forget to make time for each other and begin to grow apart through mutual neglect, your child will sense your distance and suffer for that knowledge. Don't ever forget, you and your lover are your child's primary role models for what a healthy and loving relationship is.

This ritual is designed to help you make a special commitment to each other in which you will always put the relationship, and each other, first. This does not mean that you will wait to take your child to the doctor because you have plans to go to a movie. But it does mean that you won't forget you are sensual, sexual adults. You are more than parents. You are lovers. And because you are lovers you produced this child.

I recommend performing this ritual six weeks before your expected due date.

Preparing for a Child Ceremony

You will need: a pink candle, love altar

When you are ready to begin, follow these steps:

1. Create the sacred space around your love altar.

2. Invite Demeter to join you by saying:

   "Lady Demeter, we ask you to join us today to witness our rite as we declare our promise to keep our relationship sacred and foremost in our lives. We ask you to bless us with your powers of love."

3. Light the pink candle.

4. Join hands and state your vows to each other. For example:

   "(Name), darling, I swear to you that I will keep our love sacred. I will never forget all you mean to me, no matter how much our lives change. I promise to devote time to you, and only to you, each and every day for the rest of our lives."

   Or, "(Name), sweetie, I promise to keep our love in my heart and renew it daily through my thoughts and actions. I will make time for you, and only to you, each and every day for the rest of our lives."

5. Both of you place your hands on the mother's pregnant belly, directing your attention to the child inside. Make vows to the baby, using words such as:

   "Sweet child, never fear that we don't love you when we desire time alone with each other. That time will strengthen our bond and make our union safe."

6. Say, *"I love you,"* to each other and to your child.

7. Thank Demeter for joining you:

   "Lady Demeter, we thank you for witnessing our rite and blessing us with your powers of love. We will hold our words sacred always. Farewell and blessed be."

8. Release your sacred space.

9. After you are out of sacred space, reaffirm your vows by cuddling and comforting one another. Because of the nearing due date, you may not be comfortable making love, but celebrate your promises to each other in other ways.

10. Try to recall these vows during times when you have become completely absorbed in parenthood and then try to remedy the situation with your lover at the next available opportunity.

Part Four

Healing & Banishing Rituals

We all hope our relationships will be perfect, but the truth is, they never will be. Each of us is human, we know how to hurt each other, and sometimes we do just that. That is one of the risks of love. Pain can also come from external forces, but hopefully our lovers are there to support us and help us through the difficult times.

The rituals that follow are designed to heal the hurts with our lovers. They will also help solve relationship problems or help to remove external forces that can interfere with an otherwise healthy relationship.

To continue to grow and thrive, you must let go of the pain, no matter how hard it is to do so. I hope these rituals will help you let the hurt go, let the love in, and let the healing begin.

Chapter 26

RELEASING FESTERING NEGATIVITY

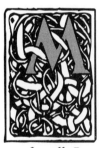y lover and I both know how to hold a grudge and so sometimes when we fight, past hurts are dredged back up and the old wounds open again. I devised this ritual to heal these emotional injuries once and for all. It can be performed in combination with any of the previous rituals, or by itself. Before you begin, both you and your lover must be willing to get rid of the grudge, let go of the pain, and stop using it as a shield against each other. It's not easy to let go of issues over which we feel deeply wronged, but if we don't, they fester and become blackened sores that infect everything else in the relationship.

For this ritual you will need the love body wash (see page 9.) You are literally going to wash the pain away from each other. If you haven't already made some, do so now, or purchase a lavender body wash. I recommend using a high-quality product that contains natural lavender. You will probably also want to buy a special bath puff for this ritual. A pink one is recommended, but white or blue will do the job.

This ritual is best performed at night when you are guaranteed time alone in the bathroom. I prefer doing it in the shower, but a bathtub will work equally well.

Prior to the ritual, arrange the candles in the room and light them. Fill the tub with comfortably warm water or warm up the shower.

Releasing Festering Negativity Ritual

You will need: a bath puff, love body wash, bath or shower, lots of pink candles

When you are ready to begin, remove each other's clothes, then follow these steps:

1. Create sacred space in the bathroom.

2. Invite Brighid to join you by saying:

   "Lady Brighid, goddess of healing, please join us as we prepare to wash away the negative feelings that linger so that they no longer bring us harm."

3. Step into the tub or shower. Using liberal amounts of body wash, gently wash each other from head to toe, one person at a time. While you do this, imagine that all of your lover's negative feelings, past hurts, and lingering pain are being rinsed away. While you are being cleansed, let all those

pent-up grudges and resentful thoughts and doubts drain away. Let it wash out of your body to make room for new feelings.

4. When you both feel cleansed and renewed, say:

"Lady Brighid, we are cleansed and purified. No longer will these pains fester between us. Please bless us with purity and renewed love."

5. Come together in the Tantric sitting position if you can do this comfortably. If not, stand together, chest-to-chest, belly-to-belly, arms around each other. Caress, kiss, and whisper, *"I love you."*

6. When you feel recharged and in love again, thank Brighid for joining you:

"Lady Brighid, goddess of healing, we thank you for helping us heal. We are honored by your gifts. Stay if you will, go if you must. Farewell and blessed be."

7. Turn off the shower, step out of the tub. Gently dry each other off with thick, luxurious towels.

8. Release your sacred space.

9. Go into the bedroom and make love to express your renewed devotion.

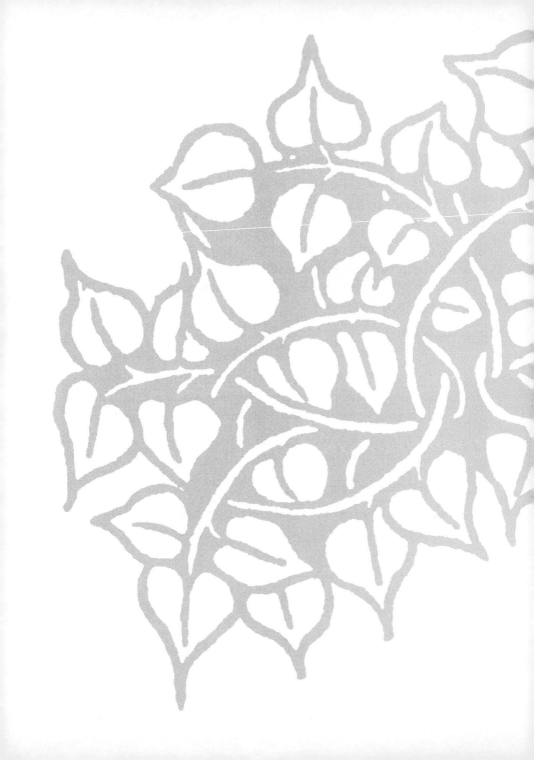

Chapter 27

CLEANSING YOUR RELATIONSHIP

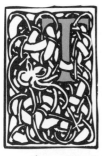his ritual is an alternative to the releasing festering negativity ritual on page 105. It's especially useful if you know the exact cause of your pain or anger. It's also good to give your relationship a periodic cleansing, just like spring cleaning in your home. Sometimes we have cobwebs we don't even know about until we go poking around in dark corners and something scary jumps out. Better to do a thorough cleaning before it has a chance to start weaving an entangling web.

Before you begin, find something in your home that reminds you of a particularly bad fight or difficult time. It should be flammable and small enough to burn in a cauldron (or you can do this at the barbecue or fireplace), or a piece of parchment paper will be sufficient.

Cleansing Your Relationship Ritual

You will need: a cauldron or flame-resistant container, an item for ritual burning, or parchment paper and a pen

When you are ready to begin, follow these steps:

1. Create sacred space.

2. Invite the goddess to join you by saying:

   "O great goddess, please join us as we purge our relationship of past pain. Please help us to release this hurt and build a stronger, happier relationship."

3. Pick up the ritual item, or write a description of the fight or the hurt on the parchment paper. If you can't think of anything specific, write "All negative feelings I may not be aware of."

4. Couple-breathe and eye-gaze as you pour all of your memories of emotional pain and negativity into the ritual item or onto the parchment.

5. When you feel the item is full, place it in the cauldron. Light it on fire and say:

   "As the (item) burns, so burns the hurt that accompanied it. Lady, please take this pain from us and replace it with love."

6. Feel the pain leaving you. When the ritual item or parchment is completely burned to ash, know your pain is gone. Say:

   "Lady, our hurt is gone. This pain is healed. We are renewed. Thank you."

7. Couple-breathe and eye-gaze to raise fresh love energy. Kiss and cuddle if you feel like it.

8. When you feel full of new love energy, release the goddess:

   "O great goddess, thank you for joining us as we purged our relationship of past pain and for helping us to release this hurt. We are blessed by your guidance, as is our relationship. Stay if you will, go if you must. Farewell and blessed be."

9. Release your sacred space.

Chapter 28

HEALING A RIFT

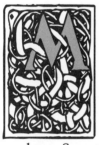

M y lover and I are passionate people, and therefore we occasionally have passionate fights. Although usually the result of a simple misunderstanding, once the fight starts, it may not end until we both feel deeply hurt. Sometimes comforting and apologizing are enough to ease the suffering; other times we need to do a little more. While this ritual won't heal every issue, it will help with many of them.

If a serious issue threatens your relationship, consider seeking professional help from a licensed therapist or couples counselor and use this ritual as part of your treatment. If you are already in therapy, I recommend this ritual as a supplement.

The ritual will work only if both of you are committed to healing the fracture and re-establishing the connection between you. You must both be ready to release each other from any blame, and you must both agree to let go of your anger and tensions before you come into the circle together. No yelling is allowed inside the circle. If this is going to be difficult, go into another room and squeeze a towel until you have literally "wrung out" your anger. Then you may return to your lover in the other room and begin.

If you want to use a special altar for this ritual, it should be a simple one with only a pink candle, perhaps a rose, and some love oil.

Healing a Rift Ritual

You will need: love oil, a pink candle, gratitude lists

Take a soothing bath to help wash away any negative thoughts. Then, follow these steps:

1. Come into the ritual naked. This symbolizes your openness to the magic and your willingness to be vulnerable.

2. Create sacred space.

3. Dress the candle with love oil by stroking the oil onto the candle from the top down to the middle and then from the bottom up to the middle. Light the candle.

4. Ask Aphrodite or your personal goddess to come to you by saying:

   "Lady Aphrodite, please join us in our healing rite. Fill us with love energy that we may work through this pain."

5. Now sit cross-legged inside the circle facing each other. Hold hands and look deeply into each other's eyes. Recall out loud why you love each other.

6. Explain why you feel hurt. Your lover should repeat the hurt back to you in his or her own words. Now your lover explains why he or she feels hurt and you repeat it back.

7. Say in unison:

   "I'm sorry."

8. Accept your lover's apology without conditions and with complete forgiveness.

9. Come into the Tantric sitting position. Couple-breathe and eye-gaze as you quietly hold each other and draw love energy in towards you. Try to feel the connection between your heart chakras by imagining a beam of light traveling between them.

10. Slowly begin to make love. Do all the things you know your lover likes, and your lover should respond in kind. This is not about great passion, although the leisurely pace will most certainly result in incredibly passionate intercourse. This is about great love and great forgiveness. By being tender with each other, you are showing your love and forgiveness in a way mere words could not.

11. After you have reached orgasm and recovered, thank Aphrodite for her assistance by saying:

    "Lady Aphrodite, thank you for joining us and lending us your energy so that we could heal our pain. This hurt is gone. Stay if you will, go if you must. Farewell and blessed be."

12. Release your sacred space.

13. Spend the rest of the night cuddling and comforting each other, then forget about this fight.

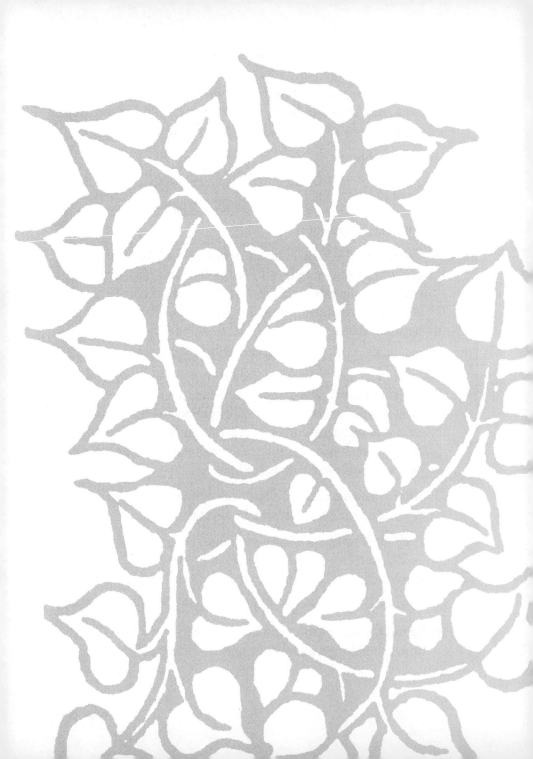

Chapter 29

RETURNING BALANCE
TO THE RELATIONSHIP

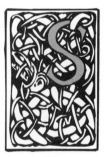

oon after my lover and I started dating, he got a job
that required him to work late at night. His schedule
severely cut into our time together and I hated it. So
I devised this ritual to help us get through that difficult period of time and restore the balance and synchronicity to
our relationship.

Once again, you will be returning to your gratitude lists for
this ritual. Review them before you begin. Also, take another look
at your vows. Are you and your lover keeping all your promises?
Are you still doing those things for each other that you used to be
grateful for? Probably not. And that's your first problem. You
have now entered the comfort stage in your relationship.

Comfort is good—and bad. It's wonderful not to worry
about getting a date for Saturday night or who will bring you soup

when you're sick. But comfort also allows you to become settled, to take each other for granted, to stop trying when it really counts. Too much comfort can slowly eat away at even the most solid relationship. Have you stopped trying to surprise each other? Stopped trying to please each other? You must start trying again!

Before you begin, each of you should think of three things you would like your lover to do that would help restore balance in your relationship. For example, if you are getting up early every morning to do something that benefits you both, ask your lover to shoulder some of the responsibility. By the same token, think of three things that you can do for your lover.

Returning Balance to the Relationship Ritual

You will need: a pink candle, parchment paper, a red pen, love oil

When you are ready to begin, follow these steps:

1. Create sacred space around you and your love altar.

2. Light your pink candle.

3. Invite Aphrodite to attend your ritual, or another goddess if you prefer. Say:

   "Lady Aphrodite, goddess of romance and relationships, please join us as we restore the balance in our relationship. Help us to keep the promises we are about to make."

4. Take turns listing the three things you would like the other to do more of, followed by the three things you each think you should be doing. All together, there should be six suggestions for each of you.

5. Write them down on a piece of parchment using a red pen. Seal the parchment by drawing the love symbol on your paper in love oil.

6. Ask Aphrodite to empower the list to ensure that balance is restored:

   "Lady Aphrodite, we ask you to bless this promise list to ensure the restoration of balance in our relationship."

7. Join hands, eye-gaze, and couple-breathe to raise energy. Focus your thoughts on restoring balance. When you feel the energy has reached a high point say in unison:

   "Our relationship is balanced."

8. Thank Aphrodite for her help:

   "Lady Aphrodite, thank you for your help in our rite. Thank you for helping us to restore the balance between us."

9. Close your sacred space. Leave the parchment paper on the altar as a reminder. But don't flaunt it. If your lover forgets, remind him or her nicely, but don't pick up the paper and point to it saying, "You said you'd do this." Guilt and accusations do nothing to restore or maintain balance in a relationship. And don't withhold your promises or affection because your lover forgot to do something. Always do your best to fulfill your promises.

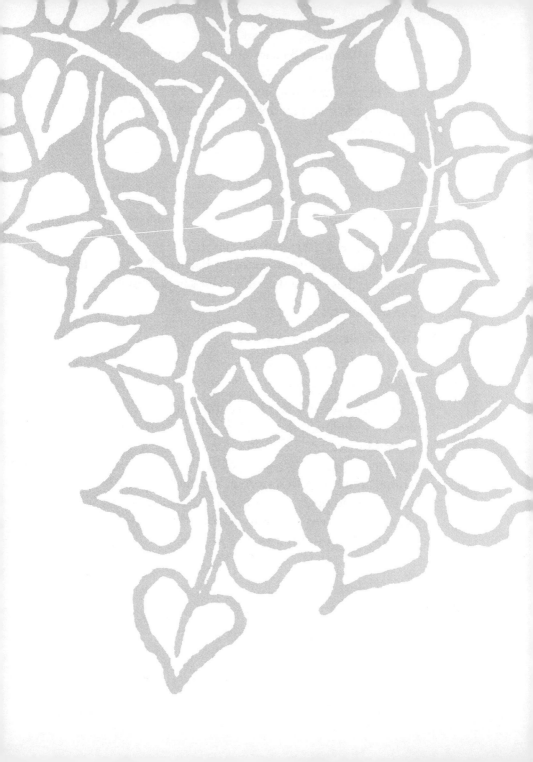

Chapter 30

BANISHING CODEPENDENCE

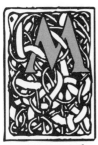y lover and I have a saying that we apply to our relationship: *"Want, not need."* This means that while we *want* to be together, we don't *need* to be together. We *want* each other, but we don't *need* each other. Of course, there are times when we do need each other for support or assistance, and that's okay. But if we were to break up, we would be able to go on with our lives. We're not so emotionally crippled that we can't function without each other, nor are we totally dependent on one another for happiness.

I have another saying: *"I make me happy."* Meaning I don't count on anyone else to provide me with the joy in my life. Only I can make me happy. Although sometimes it feels like our lovers are responsible for our happiness, in reality, it is our reaction to them that makes us happy. If someone you hated arranged to take you out for a romantic evening, it wouldn't make you happy, would it?

All that said, I know it can be a short walk from lovingly attached to being codependent. To become totally enveloped in each other, to be everything and everyone for each other, to do everything together all the time, is a romantic idea, but it's harmful to both of you. And once a codependent tendency takes hold, it's not always easy to just pull apart the strings. The next ritual can help you separate yourself from your lover if you have become codependent or feel that you are starting to become so.

For this ritual to be effective, you both need to understand that you can be together without being merged as one with each other. You will have two cords binding your wrists together. The red one is a symbol of the healthy love you share. I use red rather than pink, because red is a stronger color, and this ritual needs strength. The black cord symbolizes the unhealthy emotions that bind you together. Trust that even though you are cutting the black cord, you are *not* ending your love.

Banishing Codependence Ritual

You will need: red cord, black cord, a black candle, scissors, a cauldron or access to a fireplace

When you are ready to begin, follow these steps:

1. Create sacred space anywhere except the bedroom.

2. Invite Hecate to join you by saying:

"O great dark goddess Hecate, Goddess of purification and renewal, we ask that you join us as we remove the unhealthy ties that bind us and purify our love that it may be renewed."

3. Light the black candle.

4. Tie a knot in the red cord to make a circle, then wrap it around one of your wrists and one of your lover's wrists, saying:

   "This cord is a symbol of the healthy love we share. This relationship is our choice, not our chain."

5. Wrap the black cord around the same wrists, saying:

   "This cord is a symbol of the unhealthy ties that bind us. We wish to rid ourselves of this weight so that our relationship may once again flourish."

6. Join hands, eye-gaze, and couple-breathe to raise energy. Visualize yourselves in a healthy, happy relationship. Try to remember and recall out loud what your relationship was like before you became codependent. Know that it will be so again.

7. When you are ready, pick up the scissors. Your lover places his or her hand on top of yours. Hold the scissors over the cord and say:

   "When this cord is cut, the unhealthy ties that bind us will release us. We sever this cord, but we do not sever our love."

8. Cut the cord together. Toss it into the cauldron or fireplace and set it on alight. As it burns, feel your negative desires and needs dissipating. Know that once the cord is ash, your codependence is gone.

9. Now all that remains is the red cord. Say:

"Our love is renewed, our relationship is refreshed. 'Want, not need' shall be our oath forevermore."

10. Kiss to seal the promise.

11. Thank Hecate for her assistance by saying,

"Goddess Hecate, goddess of purification and renewal, thank you for reaffirming our love and freeing us from the dark bonds that held us. Farewell and blessed be."

9. Slip your hands out of the pink cord, leaving it tied. Release your sacred space.

10. Allow the black candle to burn all the way down. When it has extinguished itself, light the pink candle on your love altar to charge up the room. Set the red cord on your love altar.

Chapter 31

BANISHING INTERFERENCE FROM OTHERS

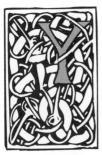ou and your lover are happily reveling in your relationship, when an ex-lover shows up wanting you or your lover back, or a friend tries to come between you out of a misguided sense of protection or jealousy. We don't always know why our family, friends, or colleagues sometimes want us to end our relationships, but if you feel the desire is unwarranted, there is a way to banish the behavior—but not the person—from interfering with your relationship. However, in an extreme case it may be necessary to banish the person altogether from your lives. Please consider the consequences carefully before taking this step.

This ritual should be used as a last resort after you have exhausted all other solutions. Simply and directly asking the person to stop interfering is the most obvious course of action. Also, be sure to ask why because there may be valid reasons for their negative perception of your relationship. Consider performing the banishing codependence ritual, before moving on to this one.

If you feel that you have no alternative other than binding the person from interfering again, then continue reading.

Banishing Interference from Others Ritual

You will need: a black film canister, water, a small piece of parchment paper, a black pen, a black candle

If you are certain you want to go through with this ritual, follow these steps:

1. Create sacred space anywhere except the bedroom.

2. Invite Hecate to join you by saying:

   "Dark Hecate, goddess of protection, please join us as we bind (name) from bringing further harm to our relationship. We ask this for the good of all. And it harm none."

3. Light the black candle.

4. Visualize the person you are binding. Recall the things that were said or done to interfere with your relationship.

5. Write the person's name on the parchment with the black pen. You have two choices here. If your intention is to banish this person from your lives, imagine him or her no longer being around you. Say:

"(Name) we bind you from bringing harm to our relationship. We ask that you no longer interfere with us, that you are no longer a part of our lives. We ask that this is so for the good of all. May it bring no harm to us or to you."

If you only wish to stop the interfering behavior and retain your relationship with that person, imagine simply that the interference has stopped. Say:

"(Name), we bind you from bringing harm to our relationship. We ask that you no longer try to come between us, but remain a part of our lives. We ask this for the good of all. May it bring no harm to us or to you."

6. Place the parchment paper in the film canister and fill it two-thirds full with water. Seal the lid on the canister.

7. Hold the canister between you and your lover, eye-gaze and couple-breathe while you visualize a return to happy, unfettered days and know that the interference will stop.

    When you feel that the banishing is complete, set the canister down and say:

    "This rite is done. (Name) is bound. For the good of all, and it harm none, so mote it be."

8. Thank Hecate for her assistance:

    "Lady Hecate, great dark goddess, thank you for joining us in our rite, and helping us to protect ourselves and our relationship from harm. Farewell and blessed be."

9. Release sacred space.

10. Place the canister in the back of your freezer. Allow the candle to burn itself out.

11. If you come to a point where you wish to unbind the person, simply remove the canister from the freezer, remove the lid, and say:

"(Name) you are freed from your bonds. Go in peace."

12. Set the canister upside down in your sink so the contents will melt and wash away. If the parchment hasn't disintegrated, let it dry out, then burn it.

Chapter 32

HEALING FROM A LOSS

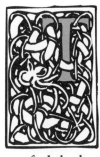he rituals in this chapter will help heal a major loss such as the death of a pet, a child, a friend, or a family member. Losing your job can also bring on a state of mourning. In some of these cases, one of you may feel the loss more strongly. In this case, the person who is feeling the loss less acutely should provide comfort and support for the more bereaved partner.

When you are both dealing with a personal loss, allow yourselves time to grieve separately, taking turns being supportive to one another. If you reach a point where one or both of you is emotionally blocked, the following ritual may help release that block and return you to the functioning world, although it will not rid you of your grief entirely.

Several years ago I lost my beloved aunt. Utterly grief-stricken, I became emotionally numb and unable to function. Once I reawakened my emotions, I was better able to get through the day and, eventually, say goodbye to my aunt.

Although this ritual involves making love, orgasm is not the goal. The intention is to awaken the deep physical sensations to which your primal emotional experiences are attached. This helps to reawaken your ability to wade through your grief and release it. By making love with your lover, you are also reminded of the love and support you already have to help you get through this difficult time.

Prior to performing the ritual, you may wish to make an altar to honor the deceased. Place favorite objects, mementos, and foods on the altar along with a photo of the departed. Perform the ritual at this special commemorative altar.

Healing from a Loss Ritual

You will need: a black candle, mementos and a photo of the departed

When you are ready to begin, follow these steps:

1. Create sacred space around your entire home.

2. Invite Persephone to join you by saying:

   "Lady Persephone, queen of the dead, please join me as I say goodbye to the one I lost. Please help me find peace once again."

3. Light a black candle for your loss and place the memento of the person or situation on the altar or somewhere nearby if you haven't made one. As you watch the candle burn, say goodbye and ask the goddess to bring you peace.

4. Without closing the circle, adjourn to the bedroom. Take time to comfort each other if you are both grieving, or the nongrieving lover should comfort the grieving lover.

5. Now begin to make love at an easy pace. Take it slowly. Don't worry about doing it "right." Just go with the sensations and see where they take you. Open yourself up to the experience. Allow the feelings to wash over you. If you are the nongrieving partner, focus on reawakening sensation in your lover. Don't be surprised if this experience manifests powerful emotional responses, such as crying or screaming.

6. Once your lovemaking has subsided, whether or not one or both of you have reached orgasm, lie together quietly, cuddling and comforting each other.

7. When you feel ready, release the goddess:

   "Lady Persephone, queen of the dead, thank you for helping me to say goodbye and helping me find peace with my loss. Farewell and blessed be."

8. Release your sacred space.

9. It will take more time before you feel normal again. This is okay. Just remember that your lover is there to support you.

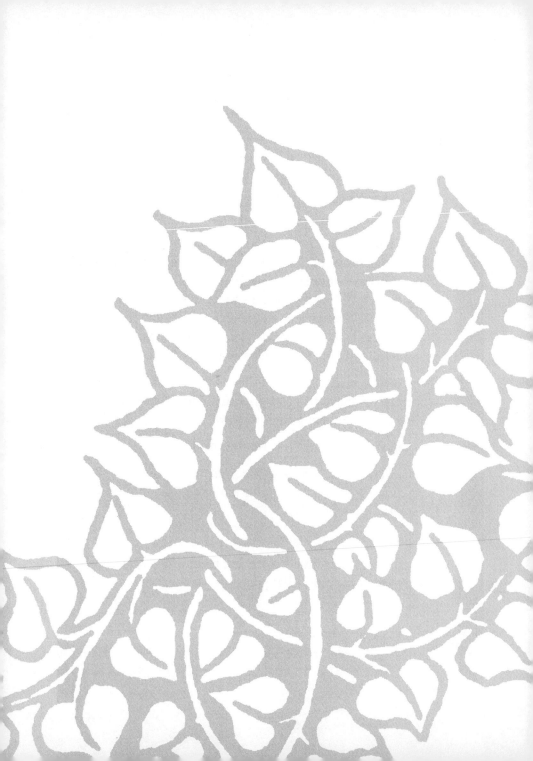

Chapter 33

HEALING SEXUAL PROBLEMS

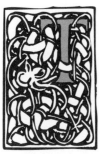here are as many attitudes towards sex as there are people on the planet. And sad to say, some of these attitudes cause needless suffering, including inhibited desire, shame about our preferences, embarrassment about our bodies, and fear of the emotional intimacy that accompanies physical intimacy. To help cope with some of these issues, I have found that ritual massage and relaxation techniques can be extremely effective. A basic, gentle massage will relax and revive a tired, stressed-out lover. It can be a prelude to intercourse, or just a loving gift.

There is also a form of massage that is expressly for pleasuring. It is basically foreplay that does not necessarily culminate with intercourse and orgasm. Pleasuring for its own sake helps you celebrate your relationship by lavishing time and attention on each other, without the pressure of "achieving" anything.

If you have fallen into a pattern of going straight for the same familiar erogenous zones on each other's bodies, impose a ban on those parts during your pleasuring session. Your skin is the largest sexual organ on your body and you'd be surprised how much of it we tend to forget or ignore, like the soles of the feet, the backs of the knees, the insides of the elbows, the palms of the hands, the back of the neck. Make it a point to touch each one of these spots next time you pleasure your lover and see what happens. Massage can also be incorporated into the Tantric sitting position by running your hands, your lips, and even your hair over each other's skin as you rock in each other's arms.

Massage can be performed within your sacred space or in conjunction with any healing ritual. But the healing sexual problems ritual that follows on pages 141–42 was designed to be used with the yoni and lingam massages on pages 135–41. These techniques were developed by Jeffery Tye and incorporate Tantric concepts. The original articles appear on Tantra.org. Please read his instructions carefully before performing the ritual.

I recommend that you only do one massage per night. Your lover may be too emotionally wrung out to return the favor after an especially intense session. Also, it may take several massages to fully release an issue. If this is the case, try not to block yourself from the emotional catharsis you felt the first time. Trust that your lover is there to protect and support you and let the emotions come out as they will.

The Yoni Massage by Jeffery Tye

Yoni (pronounced "yo-nee") is a Sanskrit word for the vagina that is loosely translated as "Sacred Space" or "Sacred Temple." In Tantric tradition, the yoni is seen from a perspective of love and respect. This is especially helpful for men to learn.

The purpose of the yoni massage is to create a space for the woman (the receiver) to relax, enter a state of high arousal, and experience pleasure from her body. Her partner (the giver) experiences the joy of being of service and witnessing a special moment. The yoni massage is an excellent activity for building trust and intimacy.

The goal of the yoni massage is not orgasm, although this is often a pleasant and welcome side effect. The goal is simply to pleasure and massage the yoni/vagina. Thus, both receiver and giver can relax and not worry about achieving anything. Orgasm is allowed to happen or not happen. It is also helpful for the giver to not expect anything in return. Just allow the receiver to enjoy the massage and to relax into herself afterward. Of course, other sexual activity may follow, but it should be entirely the receiver's choice. This perspective will build greater intimacy and trust, and will greatly expand your sexual horizons.

Preparation: Bathing is a helpful precursor as it relaxes both the receiver and giver. Include music, candles, pillows, or whatever makes the participants feel comfortable. Allow plenty of time, so there is no need to rush through the process. Go to the bathroom beforehand to avoid interrupting the massage. Connect with your partner by hugging, holding, eye-gazing, or whatever brings you to a place of safety and relaxation.

Procedure: Have the receiver lie on her back with a pillow under her head. Place another pillow, covered with a towel, under her hips, her legs spread apart with the knees slightly bent (pillows or cushions under the knees will also help). The giver sits cross-legged between the receiver's legs on a pillow or cushion.

Before any touching begins, both giver and receiver should breath deeply and remember to keep breathing throughout the massage. The giver will gently remind the receiver to start breathing again if the receiver stops or takes shallower breaths. Deep breathing, not hyperventilating, is important here.

Begin by gently massaging the legs, abdomen, thighs, and breasts to relax the receiver. Then pour a small quantity of a high-quality oil or lubricant on the mound of the yoni. Pour just enough lubricant so that it drips down the outer lips and covers the outside area. Begin gently massaging the mound and outer lips of the yoni. Do not rush. Relax and enjoy giving the massage. Gently squeeze the outer lip between the thumb and index finger, and slide up and down the entire length of each lip. Do the same to the inner lips of the yoni. Take your time.

The receiver can massage her own breasts or just relax and continue breathing deeply. It is helpful for the giver and the receiver to look into each other's eyes. The receiver can tell the giver if the pressure, speed, and depth need to be increased or decreased, but try to limit your conversation. (In my experience, too much talking distracts the focus and diminishes the effects.)

Gently stroke the clitoris in clockwise and counter-clockwise circles. Gently squeeze it between thumb and index fingers. Do not bring the receiver to orgasm. The receiver will undoubtedly become aroused but continue to encourage her to just relax and breathe.

Slowly, and with great care, insert the middle finger of your right hand into the yoni. Gently explore and massage the inside of the yoni with this finger. Take your time, be gentle, and feel up, down and sideways. Vary the depth, speed, and pressure. Remember, this is a massage. With your palm facing up, and the middle finger inside the yoni, move the middle finger in a beckoning, "come here" gesture back toward the palm. You will contact a spongy area of tissue just under the pubic bone, behind the clitoris. This is the G-spot or in Tantra, the female "Sacred Spot." Your partner may feel as if she has to urinate or it may be painful or pleasurable. Again, vary the pressure, speed, and pattern of movement. You can move your finger side-to-side, back-and-forth, or in circles. You can also insert your ring finger, but check with your partner first. Most women will enjoy the increased stimulation from two fingers. Take your time and be very gentle.

You may use the thumb of the right hand to stimulate the clitoris as well. Another option is to insert the pinky of the right hand into her anus. Ask her first and do not insert your pinky into her vagina after it has been in her anus. Use plenty of lubricant and be gentle.

Use your left hand to massage the breasts, abdomen, or clitoris. If you massage the clitoris it's usually best to use your thumb in an up-and-down motion, with your hand resting on and massaging the mound. The dual stimulation of right and left hands is very pleasurable for the receiver. I do not recommend using your left hand to touch your own genitals, because it may take your focus off the receiver. Remember, this massage is for *her* pleasure, and much of the benefit comes from not only the physical stimulation, but the intent as well.

Continue massaging using different speeds, pressures and motions. Keep breathing and looking into each other's eyes. Powerful emotions may come up and she may cry. Just keep breathing. Be a giving, loving, and patient partner.

If she has an orgasm, keep her breathing, and continue massaging if she wants. More orgasms may occur, each gaining in intensity. In Tantra this is called "Riding the Wave." Many women learn to be multi-orgasmic with the yoni massage and a patient partner.

Keep massaging until she tells you to stop. Slowly, gently, and with respect, remove your hands. Allow her to just lie still and enjoy the afterglow. Cuddling or holding is very soothing as well.

The Lingam Massage by Jeffery Tye

The Sanskrit word for the male sexual organ is lingam (pronounced "ling-ahm") and is loosely translated as "Wand of Light." In Tantra, the lingam is respectfully viewed and honored and channels creative energy and pleasure.

The purpose of the lingam massage is to help the receiver to relax and receive expanded pleasure from his lingam. His partner (the giver) experiences the joy of facilitating and witnessing the man surrendering to his softer, gentler side. It is used to help men heal from negative sexual conditioning and trauma.

Orgasm is not the goal of the lingam massage, although it is often a pleasant and welcome side effect. The goal is to massage the lingam, the testicles, perineum, and male "Sacred Spot" (the equivalent to the female G-spot), and allow the man to surrender to a form of pleasure he may not be used to. Most men need to learn to relax and receive because traditional sexual conditioning has the man in an active, goal-oriented mode.

Preparation: Take a relaxing bath or shower. Go to the bathroom before beginning the massage. The best results occur when the bowels and bladder are empty. Let go of your thoughts and connect with your partner through hugging, holding, and eye-gazing, bringing you both to a place of relaxation and trust.

Procedure: Have the receiver lie on his back with a pillow under his head. Place another pillow, covered with a towel, under his hips, his legs spread apart with the knees slightly bent (pillows or cushions under the knees will also help). The giver sits cross-legged between the receiver's legs on a cushion. Before touching the body, begin with deep, relaxed breathing. Gently massage the legs, abdomen, thighs, chest, nipples, etc., and remind the receiver to breathe deeply.

Pour a small quantity of high-quality oil on the shaft of the lingam and testicles. Begin gently massaging the testicles, taking care to not cause pain in this sensitive area. Massage the scrotum and the area above the lingam, on the pubic bone. Massage the perineum, the area between the testicles and anus. Take your time massaging this often-neglected area of the body.

Massage the shaft of the lingam, varying the speed and pressure. Gently squeeze at the base with your right hand, pull up and slide off and then alternate with your left hand. Take your time, left, right, left, right. Then change the direction by starting the squeeze at the head of the lingam and then sliding down and off, alternating with right and left hands. Massage the head of the lingam in a twisting motion as if you are using an orange juicer.

The lingam may or may not go soft during the massage. Don't worry if it doesn't get hard again. It will probably get hard, then go soft, get hard again, and so on, which is a highly desirable experience in Tantric terms. If it appears that the receiver is going to ejaculate, back off, allowing the lingam to soften a little before resuming the massage. Do this several times, coming close to ejaculation, and then backing off. Remember, the goal is not orgasm in and of itself. Deep breathing is key here and will reduce the urge to ejaculate.

There are two ways to find the male Sacred Spot. One is by locating the small indentation, about the size of a pea, midway between the testicles and anus. Gently push inward. He will feel the pressure deep inside and it may be intensely painful at first. You can massage his lingam with your right hand and massage his Sacred Spot with your left.

Another way to access the Sacred Spot is through the anus. Many heterosexual men especially are uncomfortable at first thanks to negative sexual and social conditioning. Go slowly and use plenty of lubricant. Make sure he is breathing deeply as you slip a finger into the anus, about an inch or so. Then crook the finger in a beckoning "come here" gesture. You will feel the prostate gland. Vary the pressure and speed of the massage. He may want stimulation of the lingam as you massage the Sacred Spot. Back off on the lingam as he approaches orgasm and increase the pressure on the Sacred Spot.

Powerful emotions may come up during this process. You (the giver) have created a place of trust and intimacy, so allow him to experience his feelings. Encourage him to scream, cry, moan, or sob—whatever feels appropriate. Be the best friend and healer he could have in that moment.

If he chooses to ejaculate, encourage him to breathe deeply during the orgasm. It will blow his mind, especially if he has come close and held back several times before ejaculating.

When he feels complete with the massage, gently remove your hands and allow him to lie quietly. You may want to snuggle up together or you can leave the room and let him drift off into a meditative state or sleep.

Healing Sexual Problems Ritual

You will need: a comfortable setting, a soft blanket, pillows, lubricant

Follow the preparatory suggestions above, such as bathing and going to the bathroom. Then follow these steps:

1. Create sacred space around the area where you will give the massage.

2. Invite the goddess to join you for the yoni massage, the god for the lingam massage by saying:

   "Goddess, mother of all, (or god, father of all,) please join us as we participate in the yoni (lingam) massage. Help us to release sexual pain and expand our sexual pleasure."

3. Begin with hugging, couple-breathing, and eye-gazing to establish your connection.

4. Now the giver and receiver should get into their respective positions as described above. If you are the receiver, relax. Allow any emotions that come up to be released. Do not censor yourself. You may laugh, cry, scream, shiver, or have an orgasm. Try not to stop the first painful emotion that comes up. Continue the massage until you have worked through it, unless you absolutely can't. Then stop. Don't injure yourself by pushing too far.

5. After the massage, make love if you wish, or simply lie back and relax.

6. Release the goddess or god:

"Goddess, mother of all, thank you for your assistance in this healing. My sexual nature is an honor to you."

7. Release your sacred space.

Chapter 34

STRESS BREAK BOX

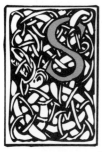

tress can be a relationship nightmare, often leading to stupid fights that can tear a relationship apart. This ritual is most useful for the smaller stresses that may result from external sources. Deeper relationship issues may be addressed by employing the releasing stress ritual on pages 148–49. The stress break box is more helpful for minor matters that can safely be set aside for a short period of time.

Before you begin, you need a box of any size. Paint it black, inside and out, or buy a box that is already black. You might also wish to place a black onyx stone inside the box. If you use a crystal, cleanse it every three months or so by soaking it in rock salt for three days. Keep parchment paper and a black pen near the box for easy access. If you run out of parchment paper, use regular paper (to avoid stressing out over something else!). If you like, place a bill in your box, (but make a note of the due date so you don't forget to pay it!).

After the initial blessing, there's no need for a formal ritual every time you place a stress in the box. Just write the stress on the parchment paper, place it inside, and say: *"Goddess, relieve me of this stress until I can deal with it."* Then forget about it until you are able to resolve the stressor.

When you are ready to deal with the problem, take the stress out of the box and read it again. If you can solve it, then do so. Burn the paper after the problem has been solved. If the problem cannot be solved, then there's no point in stressing over it anymore. Burn the paper. If you've decided there's no point in solving it, burn it also. As it burns, feel the stress going up in smoke. Say: *"This stress is gone. Goddess bless me."* If you are using a bill, burn a photocopy rather than the original.

Stress Break Box Ritual

You will need: a black box, a black onyx or crystal, strips of parchment paper, a black pen

When your box is ready, follow these steps to bless it:

1. Create sacred space.

2. Invite the goddess or your personal deity to join you:

   "Goddess, mother, protector, please join us as we bless this box to remove and purify the stresses of life. Please bless this box to aid us in this."

3. Hold the crystal between you. Eye-gaze and couple-breathe to raise energy. Your intention is to charge the crystal to relieve stress. When it is charged, place it in the box.

4. Place the box between you. Join hands, eye-gaze, and couple-breathe to raise more energy. Your intention is to charge the box with enough energy to hold those stresses away from you and protect you from them while they are in the box.

5. When the box is charged, say:

"This stress break box is blessed. When we have a stress, we put it in the box, and there it will stay until it can be solved. We will not worry about the issue while it is in the box. So mote it be."

6. If you have something to write down, put it in the box now.

7. Thank the goddess for her blessing:

"Goddess, mother, protector, thank you for helping us to alleviate our stress and for blessing the stress break box. We are honored by your assistance. Stay if you will, go if you must. Farewell and blessed be."

8. Release your sacred space.

9. Store the box in a closet or out of the way so you don't think about it once the stresses are contained within it. Recharge the box annually.

Chapter 35

RELEASING STRESS

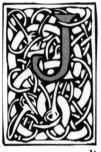

ust as there are several kinds of stress, there are several ways to release stress. This ritual is designed to come to the aid of couple or relationship stress. This kind of stress creeps up on you slowly, then suddenly pounces, digs in, and stays. It's not easy to banish it, but it feels great when you do. Relationship stress can come from diverging personal values, disagreements about money, differing family expectations, changing career goals—the list is a long one. Suffice it to say the key is to find ways to release the stress *before* it has a chance to burrow under your skin and infect your soul—and your relationship.

It's true—there's nothing like sex to relieve stress, but it's only a stop-gap solution unless it's accompanied by an honest discussion of the issue at hand. You'll need to create a safe space for this. I recommend not doing this in your bedroom in front of your love altar. A better, more neutral place would be the living room.

This ritual will encourage you to discuss the problem and air your issues, and also create a solution. There should be no judgments, no fights, no nasty words. Don't edit yourself, but don't be accusatory or demeaning. Understand that you are *both* part of the cause and *both* part of the solution. So, acknowledge each other's feelings. Listen to one another. And try to understand.

Releasing Stress Ritual

You will need: enough candles to create a circle, two pillows

When you are ready to begin, follow these steps:

1. Create a circle of candles on the floor and place two comfy pillows in the middle.

2. Create sacred space within the circle.

3. Invite the goddess to join you by saying:

   "Goddess, ruler of love, please join us as we create this safe haven that we may openly discuss our issues without fear of resentment and anger. Please bless us with your calming presence."

4. Facing each other, hold hands, eye-gaze, and couple-breathe.

5. Remind yourselves that this is a safe haven for talking. Start the discussion with:

   "I promise to listen and to do my best to understand without judging or taking offense."

It's a challenge, but you can do it.

6. Take turns speaking about whatever is causing you stress.

7. Create a solution together.

8. When you are talked out and satisfied that your solution is realistic, come into the Tantric sitting position to share a kiss.

9. Release the goddess:

   "Great goddess, ruler of all, we thank you for facilitating this process. Our love is an honor to you and your love is an honor to us. Stay if you will, go if you must. Farewell and blessed be."

10. If you feel so inclined, you can release your sacred space, move out of the circle of candles, and retreat to your bedroom to make love. Make sure you extinguish the candles before you go. There's nothing like burning down your house to create stress!

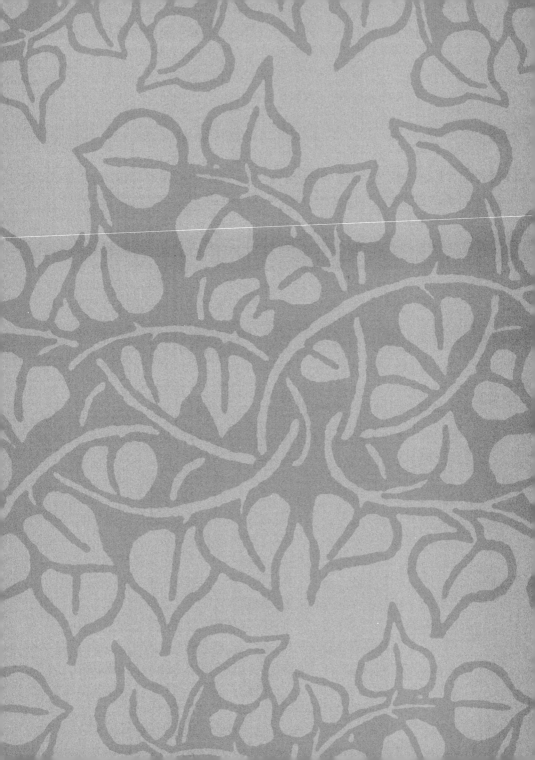

Part Five

Blessings & Manifesting Rituals

These rituals are designed to help you meet your goals, attain your desires, bless your physical surroundings, and manifest material things. They will benefit individual desires or joint goals.

My lover and I love to perform manifesting rituals. We do it all the time. Manifesting is the magical act of bringing our hearts and desires into being. Often we ask for things we feel we were meant to have anyway, but we want to accelerate the process. The gods work on a different time line than we do. Sometimes we have to remind them that we don't have a thousand years to wait.

When you perform a manifesting ritual, be careful to avoid mentioning specific people or institutions. You don't want inadvertently to manipulate someone's will. With that caveat in mind, start manifesting today!

Chapter 36

BLESSING EACH OTHER FOR LOVE

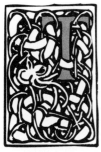his ritual was designed as a self-blessing for my work-shops, but it is even more effective when you and your lover bless each other for love. It is a gift you give to your relationship, because everything you are and everything you do is blessed with the support of your lover and the gifts of the goddess.

This ritual can be performed anytime, but I think it's best on a Friday or during the waxing moon. Take five minutes or five hours, it's entirely up to you and your partner. It can precede or follow any of the other rituals in this book.

Blessing Each Other for Love

You will need: love oil, a pink candle

When you are both ready, begin the ritual:

1. Prepare by taking a shower or relaxing bath. Wash each other's bodies slowly and lovingly, but not as a prelude to lovemaking.

2. Step out of the shower and dry each other off.

3. Create sacred space.

4. Light the pink candle. Invite Aphrodite to attend your ritual by saying:

   "Lady Aphrodite, we ask you to join us as we bless ourselves and each other with your gifts of love, joy, and sensuality, which we honor and celebrate."

5. Anoint your lover by placing a small amount of oil on your fingertips, then draw a heart on your lover's forehead.

   Say: *"I bless you with passion eternal."*

   Touch the oil to your lover's lips.

   Say: *"I bless you with poetry eternal."*

   Touch the oil to your lover's heart.

   Say: *"I bless you with love eternal."*

   Touch the oil to your lover's genitals.

   Say: *"I bless you with sensuality eternal."*

   Touch the oil to your lover's feet.

   Say: *"I bless you with support eternal."*

6. Now your lover anoints you in the same manner.

7. Then encircle one another in your arms. Share a kiss to seal the blessing. When you part, say:

   "We are blessed with the gifts of Aphrodite."

8. Release Aphrodite from your sacred space. Say:

   "Lady Aphrodite, we thank you for your gifts of love, sensuality, and joy. We will treasure and honor them eternally. Go with the peace and love in our hearts."

9. Release your sacred space.

10. Now is a great time to make love!

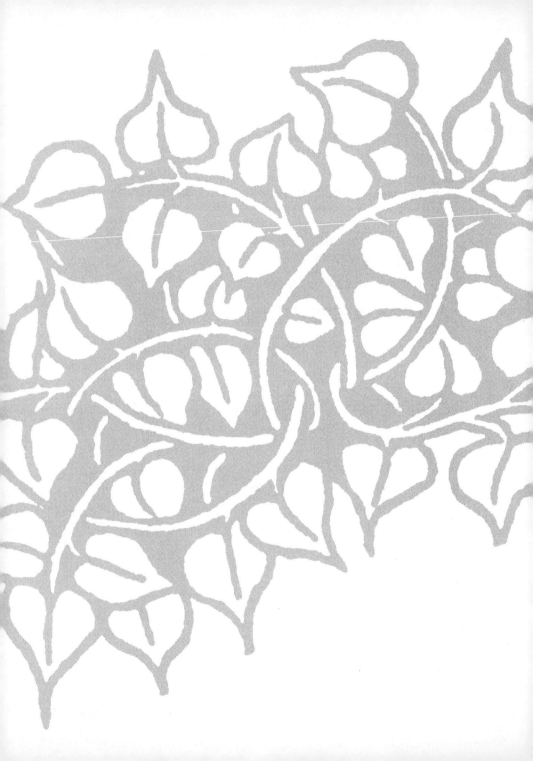

Chapter 37

BLESSING YOUR RELATIONSHIP CRYSTAL

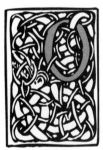

ne of the items on your love altar is a crystal that recharges and energizes your love and your relationship. When you blessed your love altar (see pages 29–31), you placed a simple blessing on the crystal. This ritual creates a more specific blessing, or you may use it to bless a second crystal to use somewhere else in your home.

Crystals not only collect energy, they reflect it, recharge it, and renew it. They can bring transformation, healing, and blessing into your home. The rose quartz crystal is an especially powerful love and relationship crystal, although its energy is very gentle and peaceful. Some crystals are cut into a heart-shape, which I find even more effective for this particular ritual. But it's fine to use any crystal, whether it's shaped or natural, polished or unpolished, that feels right to you.

You do have to be careful with crystals though. Because they both gather and amplify energy, make sure you cleanse your crystal periodically. Also, cleanse it before you perform this ritual. Set the crystal on rock salt for three days, wash it in spring water, or leave in the light of the full moon overnight.

Blessing Your Relationship Crystal

You will need: a rose quartz crystal

When your crystal is cleansed, begin the ritual:

1. Create sacred space.

2. Invite the element of earth to join you if you haven't already called the quarters. If you have, ask the element for a special blessing for your crystal by saying:

   "Element of earth, crystal spirit join us as we charge this rose quartz, your loving gift to us, to be the physical manifestation of our love."

4. Holding the crystal between you, eye-gaze and couple-breathe.

5. Feel the energy expand between you, connecting your heart centers, then flowing down into the crystal.

6. When you feel the crystal is fully charged, say:

   "This crystal holds the essence of our love. May it renew our relationship always."

7. Release the element by saying:

   "Element of earth, crystal spirit, thank you for your gift, which blesses our relationship."

8. Release your sacred space.

9. Place the crystal on your love altar, in the relationship corner of your home or bedroom, on your nightstand, or under your bed.

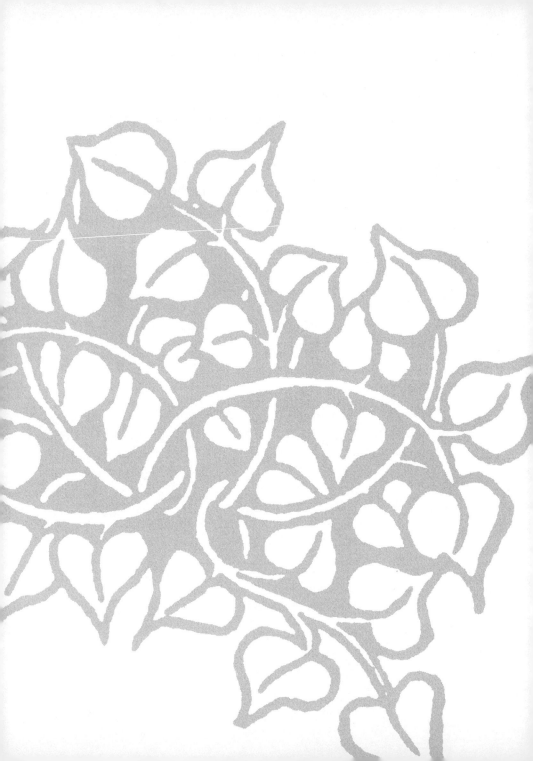

Chapter 38

BLESSING YOUR RELATIONSHIP CANDLE

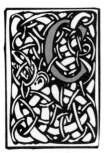

andles have a special place in my life and my home. This is a specific blessing for your relationship candle to help keep the love and romance flowing between you. Burn your relationship candle for at least fifteen minutes a minimum of once a week. (Of course, you may do this more often as you desire.) This will infuse your relationship and your home with love energy and with the powerful, passionate energy inherent in the fire element. It also unleashes the special properties contained in the love oil.

Blessing Your Relationship Candle

You will need: a pink candle, love oil

When you've gathered the supplies, begin the ritual:

1. Create sacred space.

2. Invite Aphrodite to join you by saying:

   "Lady of love, Aphrodite, we call you. Thank you for bringing love into our lives. Please join us as we bless this candle to bring our relationship eternal love."

3. Hold the candle between you as you eye-gaze and couple-breathe to raise energy. Your intention is to charge the candle with love so that it will burn with love energy each time you light it.

4. Dress the candle in love oil by drawing the oil from the bottom up to the middle and from the top down to the middle, thereby drawing in love.

5. Set the candle in a holder and say:

   "This candle is blessed. May it infuse our lives with love each time it is lit."

6. Light the candle and make passionate love.

7. Release Aphrodite.

   "Lady of love, Aphrodite, we thank you for joining us as we blessed this candle for enduring love. We are blessed and honored by your presence. Stay if you will, go if you must. Farewell and blessed be."

8. Release your sacred space.

Chapter 39

BLESSING YOUR HOME

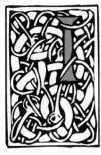t is important that you bless the space you live in. Your home is your sanctuary and should be cared for and protected. A ritual home cleansing and blessing can be performed anytime, although it is traditional to do so when you first move in. Even if you've lived in your home for many years, you can still perform an initial cleansing and blessing. It is also important to do a joint cleansing if your lover moves in with you, you move in with your lover, or you move into a new home together. Although not essential, it is ideal to perform the cleansing before you move in.

You will need white candles, candleholders, and a sage wand for each of you, or burn loose dried sage in a heat-resistant bowl and fan the smoke with a feather. When you are "smudging," as it is called, it is important that you smudge each window, door, vent, phone jack, faucet, drain, or any other opening through which energy can enter or leave your home. Smudge the interiors of your closets. Get every corner! If you live in a house, be sure to include the exterior of the building and smudge the perimeter of your property, too.

Bless each room as you enter it. For example, in your kitchen, ask the gods to bless it for good food, good drink, and much joy. Bless the living room for laughter and entertainment. Bless the office for inspiration, financial success, and peaceful working conditions. When you get to the bedroom, ask the gods to bring love, restful sleep, and great sex into the room.

Large amounts of smoke may set off your smoke alarms. Do not disable them. Think of the noise as scaring away any lingering beasties or bad energy. Don't open the windows to clear the air until the blessing is complete.

Once you have smudged your entire home, there is one more extremely enjoyable way to bless your house. We've all heard the old story about newlyweds making love in every room. Well, it's not really a joke. You should do just that. Not all on the same night, but over the course of your first month in your new place, or your first month of living together, make sure you bless each room with sexual pleasure. The energy will infuse the entire dwelling with love.

I like to re-purify my home after my lover and I have had a nasty row or worked through a serious problem.

Home Blessing

You will need: sage wands or loose sage, a bowl and a feather, white candles, several candleholders

When you are ready to begin, follow these steps:

1. Place one candle in the center of each room and light it. For safety, place each candleholder on a plate so the wax doesn't drip and start a fire. If safety is a serious concern, skip the candle entirely. I also recommend removing curious pets and small children from all areas where candles are burning unattended.

2. Invite the goddess Hestia to join you by saying:

   "Lady Hestia, protector of hearth and home, please join us as we bless our home for comfort, joy, and peace."

3. Go to the front door and light your sage wands from the candle. Make your way through your entire home, spreading the smoke in every room.

4. Bless each room as you pass through it with the activity or feeling you wish to experience there. For example, you may modify the following bedroom blessing or create your own.

   "O great goddess, bringer of all love, and from whom sexual hunger derives, please bring the joining of the two to this bed."

   Smudge the area over and around the bed especially thoroughly.

5. Return to the point where you started. Thank Hestia for her blessing.

   "Lady Hestia, protector of home and hearth, thank you for blessing our home and all who pass through it. We are

honored by your blessing. Stay if you will, go if you must. Farewell and blessed be."

6. Place your sage wands in a fireproof container to safely burn out, or carefully stub them out. Collect the candles and place them in a sink or bathtub where they can safely burn themselves out.

Chapter 40

MANIFESTING PROSPERITY AS A COUPLE

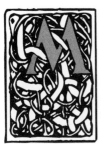y lover and I constantly worry about our finances, even though we don't need to. We're not alone in this. Money is often a key point of tension between lovers. Rather than stressing and fighting over money, work toward prosperity together. Not only will it keep the tension low, sharing a goal brings you closer together.

First, you need to agree to not keep any large purchases secret from each other. Decide ahead of time what constitutes a large purchase. Gifts are an exception, but carefully consult your budget beforehand to make sure you can afford the expense comfortably. There's no need to be stingy. Stinginess begets stinginess and generosity begets generosity. But be sensible. Also be sure to choose at least one charity to which you can make regular, affordable donations.

The blessing that follows helps to assure that you and your lover will become or remain prosperous. The box may be any size, as long as it is large enough to hold a dollar bill, and fashioned from wood, cardboard, or stone.

Prosperity Blessing

You will need: a money oil, a box, a dollar bill of any denomination, a green candle, a green pen

When you are ready to begin, follow these steps:

1. Create sacred space.

2. Invite the god and goddess of prosperity to join you in your ritual. I use Fortuna and Jupiter by saying:

   "Lady Fortuna, goddess of good fortune, please join us in this rite of prosperity. Bring us your gifts that we may grow our prosperity together as a couple. Lord Jupiter, god of prosperity, please join us in this rite of abundance. Bring us your wisdom that we may grow our prosperity together as a couple."

3. Dress the green candle with money oil, then light it.

4. Facing each other, eye-gaze and couple-breathe to raise energy.

5. When you feel that you have a strong connection and your breathing is comfortably in sync, turn to your altar. Sign your names across the bill with a green pen. Each of you should hold the bill for a moment to imbue it with your energy.

6. Place the bill in the box. Together, hold the box and say:

   "This bill is a symbol of our prosperity. May it grow and flourish as our relationship grows and flourishes. We ask that prosperity bring us together, not tear us apart. We are more than our finances. Money does not rule us."

7. Continue holding the box together or place it on the floor between you and join hands. You may need to close your eyes for this next part, but wait until you feel a strong connection and continue couple-breathing throughout. Visualize your joint prosperity. Imagine how it will feel not to fight or worry about money and how happy you will be once you have achieved your dreams.

8. When your image is complete, open your eyes. Nod to your lover as a signal that you are finished. Say in unison:

   "Prosperity is ours. This rite is done. With harm to none, so mote it be."

9. Thank the god and goddess for joining you in your ritual and for bringing you prosperity. Say:

   "Lady Fortuna, goddess of good fortune, thank you for joining us in this rite of prosperity. We are honored by your gift of prosperity. Lord Jupiter, god of prosperity, thank you for joining us in this rite of abundance. We are honored by your gift of wisdom."

10. Release your sacred space.

11. Keep the box on your love altar as a reminder of your mutual goals.

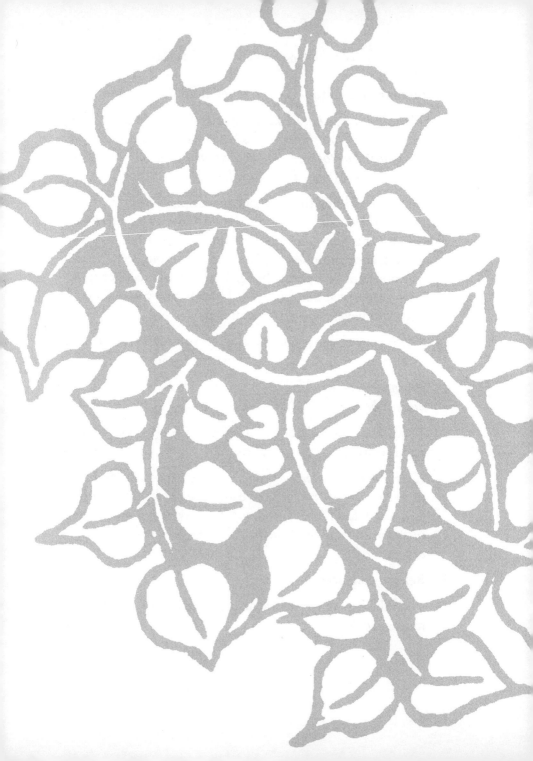

Chapter 41

MANIFESTING SPECIFIC GOALS

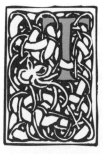his ritual is similar to the prosperity blessing, but with a few alterations. It can be used for anything you would like to manifest as a couple, including a house, a car, or a vacation. It can also be used to manifest individual desires and goals.

First you will need to choose a goddess or god to call. Examples would be Hestia for a home, Hermes for a car, and Mercury for a vacation. (See Appendix D for a list of goddesses and gods.) You will also need to find a symbol of your goal such as a miniature model house, a toy car, or travel brochures for your desired destination.

Fill in the blanks ahead of time to avoid struggling to describe your desire during the ritual. The gods don't mind the occasional stumble, giggle, or mistake, but searching for the proper phrase is too distracting.

Manifesting Specific Goals

You will need: a symbol of your goal, parchment paper, a colored pen that can write on any surface, an offering

When you are ready to begin, follow these steps:

1. Come into sacred space.

2. Invite the goddess or god you have chosen to join you by saying:

   "(Goddess or god name) please join us on this eve as we manifest our goal of (name it). Please help us to acquire what we need."

3. Facing each other, join hands, eye-gaze, and couple-breathe.

4. When you feel ready, pick up the designated symbol of your goal. Hold it in both your hands and visualize your goal. Then visualize yourselves living in your new home, driving your new car, or going on your fabulous vacation. Imagine how these things will make you feel.

5. Pick up the pen and write your full names on the symbol. If they won't fit, write your names and the goal on the parchment paper.

6. Place the symbol on your love altar (or on top of the parchment). It will remain there until you have acquired your goal.

7. Say:

   "Our goal is attained. Our desire is fulfilled. So mote it be."

8. Thank the goddess or god for his or her help in the matter.

   "Thank you (goddess or god name) for joining us, as we manifested our goal of (name it). We are honored by your assistance."

9. Release your sacred space.

10. When you acquire your goal, make some sort of offering to the goddess or god in thanks. For example, build an altar to that deity in your home, place an image in the glove compartment of your car, or sprinkle a bit of food or drink on the ground at your vacation destination.

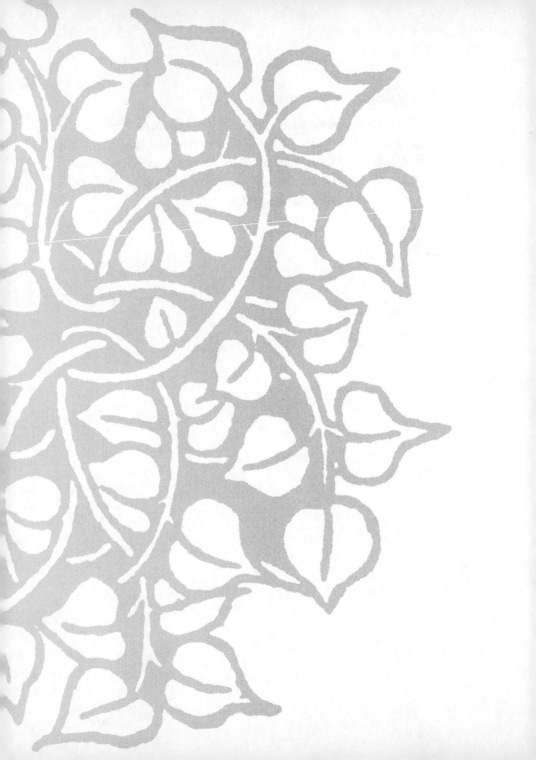

Chapter 42

MANIFESTING LONG-TERM GOALS

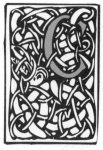ertain goals, such as the need for a job, are immediate necessities. But sometimes we have long-term objectives, such as a happy marriage or a healthy child, or even a comfortable retirement. If you and your lover share long-term goals, now is the time to plant the seeds for their growth.

You are planting both a real seed and a metaphorical seed. As the seed becomes a plant, it serves as a physical reminder of your long-term goal. You and your lover can nurture the plant the way your nurture the mutual goal, and both will be blessings on your relationship.

Planting seeds is a traditional practice for marking the spring equinox, but this ritual can be performed in any season, and on any day, although seeds generally grow better when planted during the waxing moon.

Manifesting Long-term Goals

You will need: an attractive pot or planter, potting soil, water, seeds for a plant that is suited to your region and growing space

When you have gathered your supplies, begin the ritual:

1. Decide on your joint goal.

2. Fill the pot with soil and place it on your love altar. Have everything else you will need in readiness near the pot.

3. Create sacred space.

4. Invoke the goddess that is appropriate to your goal. Popular deities include Aphrodite, Brighid, Demeter, Hestia, and Diana. Say:

   "Great goddess (name), please join us this day as we plant the seeds of growth, as we plant the seeds for continuous renewal, as we plant the seeds that are your gift to us."

5. Eye-gaze and couple-breathe to raise energy, then state your goal aloud. Say:

   "Lady (name), we ask for (goal).

6. Envision white light extending from your heart center to your lover's heart center, then extend the circle outward to include the pot and seeds.

7. Pick up the seed and hold it in your palm, filling it with your intentions. Have your lover do the same. Make a divot in the soil, place the seed inside, and gently cover it.

8. Hold the pot between you and envision your goal. Imagine how achieving it will enhance or change your relationship and your life together.

9. Pour water over the soil, dampening it slightly. Say:

   "We bless this seed to grow strong. We bless this soil to provide sustenance. We bless the two combined to bring us (state your goal). So mote it be."

10. Release the deity you invoked by saying:

    "Great goddess (name), thank you for joining us, thank you for blessing us with your presence, thank you for your gift of growth, thank you for your gift of renewal. We are honored by all you bring us. Stay if you will, go if you must. Farewell and blessed be."

11. Release your sacred space.

12. If your love altar is not in a place that will encourage the growth of a young plant, please move it somewhere where it is sure to flourish. As it grows, know that your goal is also growing.

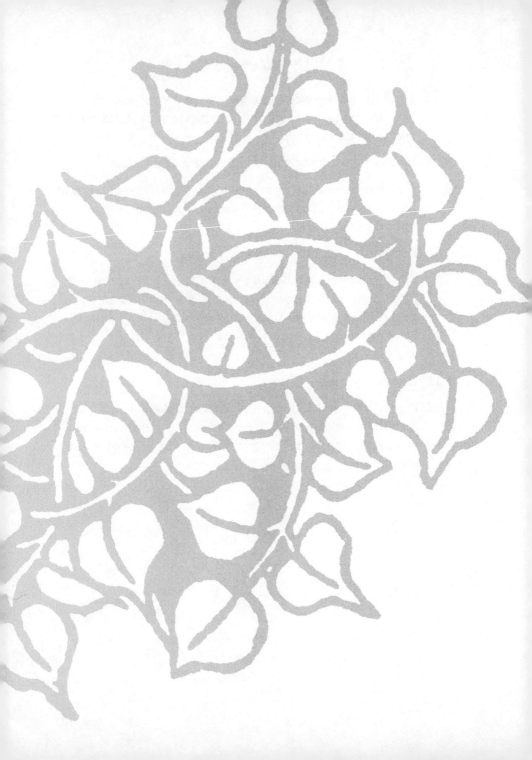

Chapter 43

MANIFESTING CAREER SUCCESS

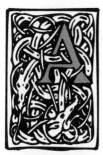lthough I try to put my relationship ahead of my career, at times I need to receive more satisfaction from my work to be happy in my relationship. Many of us define ourselves by what we do for a living. This ritual is designed to help you achieve career success, with the support of your lover, without sacrificing the relationship. It should be performed for each of you separately rather than both of you together.

Before you begin, thoughtfully determine your career goal. Be reasonable. I recommend starting with a small step or modest accomplishment, not a twenty-year achievement. For example, if you want to make senior partner at a law firm and you just graduated from law school, it would be unreasonable to expect your lover to wait for you to achieve your goal without getting some support in return. Recognize that your lover has needs that shouldn't be subjugated for yours.

If you have a favorite deity you frequently work with, call her or him. If not, you can use Jupiter, Juno, Apollo, Athena, or almost any other deity you feel comfortable with. If you work in a field that is somewhat related to a deity's area of dominion, then choose that deity. For example, writers and artists often use Brighid. A stockbroker or financial adviser might use Jupiter. A lawyer might use Athena. Computer programmers and technicians could use Jupiter, god of logic, or Mercury, god of communication.

You will also need a symbol of your career for the ritual. A pen, a picture from a magazine, a tiny charm, anything will do. As long as it has meaning for you, it will have meaning for the ritual.

Manifesting Career Success

You will need: career symbol, career deity, the support of a loving partner

When you are ready to begin, follow these steps:

1. Create sacred space.

2. Invite your deity to join you for the ritual. Personalize this invocation:

   "Lady Brighid, goddess of creativity, goddess of the pen, please join us as I seek to enhance my career. Please join us to extend your blessings over my work."

3. Take your lover's hands in yours. Promise your lover that you will not sacrifice your relationship in favor of your

career. Make two to three promises that you can keep. For example, if you are a musician, vow not to forget to call your lover when you go on tour or perform late at night. Or if you are going for a career in medicine, promise that you will make time for your lover at least once a week, no matter how time-consuming your medical residency becomes. Then keep your word!

4. The supporting lover responds with similar promises:

   "I promise to support you in your career endeavors."

   "I will understand when I have to alter social plans."

   "I will understand your efforts when they take you away from me."

5. Take turns holding the career symbol while you eye-gaze and couple-breathe. Visualize how you will feel when your lover achieves their goal with your support. Then visualize how you will feel when you are engaged in a thriving and satisfying career. Imagine how career success will enhance your relationship.

6. When you feel the symbol is charged, place it on your love altar. Or you can carry it until you have reached your goal.

7. Thank the deity you have chosen for assistance. Adapt these words:

   "Lady Brighid, goddess of creativity, goddess of the pen, thank you for assisting me with my career. We are honored by your blessings over my work."

8. Release your sacred space.

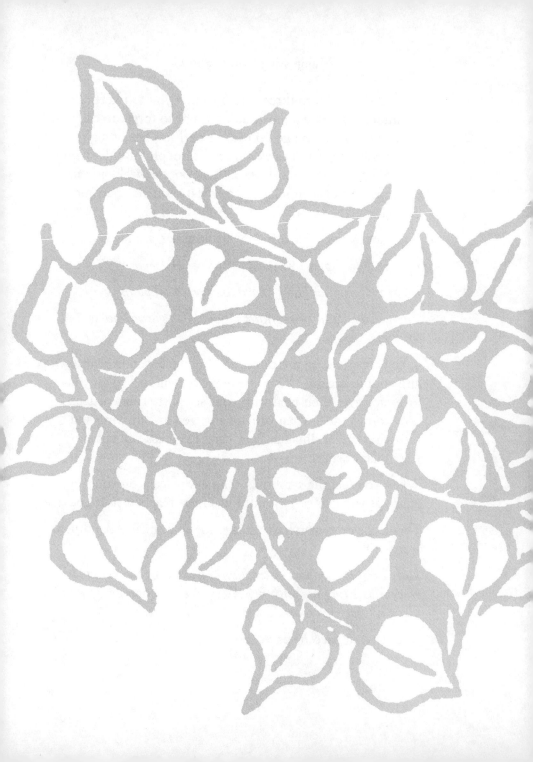

Chapter 44

CONCEIVING A CHILD

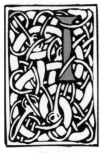 f you and your lover have decided to have a child, this ritual may help the conception process. You will need to choose a deity to call during your ritual. If you have a matron or patron you frequently work with, then by all means, call that deity. If not, Brighid, Hera, Inanna, Astarte, Demeter, Venus, and the god Min are all fertility deities.

You will need a small image or figurine of the goddess you have chosen, such as a miniature Willendorf Venus. The object should be small enough to fit in your pocket or around your neck because you will need to keep it near you until you are pregnant.

Think of a way to honor your chosen deity in return for honoring you with a child. One of my friends named her daughter after the goddess she called during her conception ritual. You might want to do the same. Or if it's an unusual name, use it as a middle name. Another idea is to place a small statue or picture of the deity in the child's room.

During the ritual, you will have an opportunity to ask for a few specific qualities, but don't go overboard. Certainly you can request a happy, healthy child. However, I wouldn't advise you to get too detailed as to eye color, hair color, height, weight, or gender.

This ceremony is best performed naked on the night of the full moon or during your most fertile period. A ritual bath or shower beforehand is recommended to prepare you and your lover emotionally and physically for this major life change.

Conception Ritual

You will need: goddess image, a white or silver candle

When you are ready to begin, follow these steps:

1. Create sacred space around your love altar and bed.

2. Invite the goddess or god you have chosen to join the ritual. Adapt these words:

   "Great mother Inanna, goddess of women and children, goddess of fertility. Please join us as we perform this ritual for conception. Please bring us your blessings, so that we may soon conceive a child to call our own."

3. Light the candle.

4. Holding the goddess image between you, promise her that you will teach the child to honor her and that you will treat the child with love always. Make any other promises you have agreed upon beforehand.

5. Request the specific qualities you desire.

6. Still holding the goddess image, eye-gaze and couple-breathe to raise the energy as you visualize having your child, how you will feel, how you will treat the child, how the child will enrich your life.

7. When the energy has reached a high point, come together in the Tantric sitting position and make love with the intention of creating a baby.

8. After you make love, thank the goddess for her assistance. Adapt these words:

   "Great mother Inanna, goddess of women and children, goddess of fertility, thank you for joining us as we performed this ritual for conception. Thank you for blessing us with a child."

9. Release your sacred space.

10. Make love as often as you feel like it. If you are the female lover, carry the goddess figure with until you conceive.

11. When your child is born, it is important to keep the promises you made during the ritual.

A FINAL NOTE

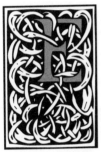very time we make love, it is a sacred act, whether or not we intend it to be. Just as the goddess has many sides, our lovemaking does, too. It is important to approach sex with the same attitude you bring to love: Sometimes it's serious, sometimes it isn't.

However, sex—even great sex—can't fix everything. You can have all the sex you want, but if your hearts aren't connecting, it's not going to make a difference. If your love is broken, no amount of sex is going to repair it. Some of the previous blessings and rituals in this book can help, but for serious problems, see a licensed therapist or couples counselor. Sometimes magic needs a little help.

Finally, don't forget to enjoy your relationship. We tend to get so caught up in the everyday events of our lives that we take our relationships and our lovers for granted. Remember that love is special. And because it is special it should celebrated and nourished. If you don't take care of it, it will languish and, eventually, it will die.

I hope the blessings and rituals in this book help you keep your love alive and flourishing. For help finding any of the products I mention, please visit my website, SeleneSilverwind.com.

May the Lady bless you with love and happiness for all your days—and nights.

Blessed be,
Selene Silverwind

Appendix A: Timing

Most of the blessings, ceremonies, and rituals in this book are best performed during the new moon, full moon, or during the waxing period in between. Rituals that manifest, create, enhance, heal, or restore are more effective during a waxing moon. Rituals that remove, banish, or release should be done during the waning period between the full and new moons. The three days prior to the new moon, the time known as the dark moon, is a particularly effective time for difficult healings and banishings. Powerful manifesting rituals, such as conceiving a child, are more effective during the full and new moons.

It's easy to keep track of these times with any calendar that indicates the lunar phases. If you are astrologically minded, avoid periods when the moon is void of course, or not "in" any astrological sign. I have found Jim Maynard's *Celestial Influences* calendar helpful in determining such times. There are also several websites that list this information. Do a search for "moon void of course" and you should find one you like.

You can also try to be aware of moon wobbles and mercury retrogrades. However, if the time feels right for the ritual, then do it. It may be almost impossible to find the "perfect" time to perform a ceremony if you're trying to squeeze it in between moon voids, mercury retrogrades, and moon wobbles. Venus also occasionally goes retrograde, so if you find yourself in real emotional trouble during these periods, try to wait them out before making any major relationship changes.

Appendix B: Days of the Week

In magical terms, each day of the week has come to be associated with certain energies and actions. These in turn are associated with the strengths and powers of the goddesses and gods each day is named for. In the English language, which evolved from Germanic and romance languages, we use the names of Teutonic and Greco-Roman deities.

So, performing a sexually enhancing ritual, such as restoring passion or creating fireworks, would be preferable on a Tuesday or Friday. However, Thursdays will be more effective for performing a manifesting ritual or blessing, such as prosperity as a couple.

These are my interpretations of these days. If you have different ideas, use yours.

Monday: *Moon's day. Intuition, women's mysteries, children, fertility, the goddess.*

Tuesday: *Tui's day. Mars. Aggression, war, passion, partnership, action, sex.*

Wednesday: *Woden's day. Mercury. Travel, writing, contracts, arts, creativity, learning.*

Thursday: *Thor's day. Jupiter. Business, politics, money, education, law, success.*

Friday: *Freya or Frigga's day. Venus. Love, friendship, beauty, harmony, marriage, sensuality.*

Saturday: *Saturn's day. Home, protection, obstacles, banishing.*

Sunday: *Sun's day. Health, career, finances, men's mysteries, creativity, the god.*

Appendix C: Color Correspondences

For magical purposes, certain colors are associated with specific actions or emotions. Again, these are the associations I prefer. Feel free to interpret your own. Use these colors to enhance your magic with candles, altar cloths, stones, and cords.

Red: *fire, strength, passion, sex, lust, swift action.*
Pink: *romantic love, family love, peace, affection, partnerships.*
Orange: *business, property, confidence.*
Yellow: *intelligence, memory, charm.*
Green: *wealth, growth.*
Blue: *creativity, tranquility, communication, health.*
Purple: *influence, spirituality, power.*
Brown: *neutrality, ending without banishing.*
Black: *banishing, protection, binding.*
White: *spirituality, peace, all-purpose.*
Gold: *the god, sun.*
Silver: *the goddess, moon, intuition.*

Appendix D: Gods and Goddesses

Throughout this book I ask you to invite Aphrodite to your ritual. I do this because the deities of Greek mythology are the most commonly recognized; however, you may substitute other goddesses or gods wherever you feel it is appropriate.

This list is by no means comprehensive. It comprises the better-known deities, along with a few obscure choices.

Aphrodite: *Greek goddess of love, beauty, and sex.*
Apollo: *Greek god of the arts.*
Astarte: *Phoenician and later Greek goddess of fertility.*
Athena: *Greek goddess of battle and protection.*
Brighid: *Celtic goddess of smithcraft, inspiration, healing, fertility, poetry, and learning.*
Cernunnos: *Celtic god of fertility.*
Demeter: *Greek goddess of motherhood and fertility.*
Epona: *Celtic goddess of fertility, prosperity, and maternity.*
Eros: *Greek god of love.*
Fortuna: *Roman goddess of good fortune and happiness.*
Frey: *Scandinavian god of fertility and abundance*
Freya/Frigga: *Scandinavian goddess of love and beauty*
Frey: *Scandinavian god of love.*
Hathor: *Egyptian goddess of motherhood.*
Hecate: *Greek goddess of the crossroads and protection.*

Hera: *Greek goddess of marriage and home.*

Hermes: *Greek god of travel, commerce, and communication.*

Hestia: *Greek goddess of hearth and home.*

Hymen: *Greek god of marriage and commitment.*

Inanna: *Sumerian mother goddess.*

Ishtar: *Sumerian goddess of sexuality and love.*

Isis: *Egyptian great mother goddess.*

Juno: *Roman goddess of home and marriage.*

Jupiter: *Roman ruler god of business, logic, and power.*

Kwan Yin: *Chinese goddess of fertility and healing.*

Mercury: *Roman god of travel, commerce, and communication.*

Min: *Egyptian god of fertility.*

Pan: *Greek god of nature and passion.*

Persephone: *Greek goddess of the underworld.*

Rosmerta: *Celtic goddess of prosperity.*

Shakti: *Hindu mother goddess, inseparable from Shiva.*

Shiva: *Hindu god of destruction, inseparable from Shakti.*

Venus: *Roman goddess of love, beauty, and sex.*

Bibliography

Budapest, Zsuzsanna. *The Goddess in the Bedroom.* San Francisco, CA: HarperSanFrancisco, 1995

Carter, Karen Rauch. *Move Your Stuff, Change Your Life.* New York, NY: Simon & Schuster, 2000.

Cunningham, Scott. *The Complete Book of Incenses, Oils, and Brews.* St. Paul, MN: Llewellyn Publications, 1996.

Cunningham, Scott. *Wicca: A Guide for the Solitary Practitioner.* St. Paul, MN: Llewellyn Publications, 1992

Dixon-Kennedy, Mike. *Celtic Myth & Legend.* London, UK: Blandford, 1996.

Hamilton, Edith. *Mythology.* New York, NY: Penguin Group, 1942.

Judith, Anodea and Selene Vega. *The Sevenfold Journey: Reclaiming Mind, Body & Spirit Through the Chakras.* Freedom, CA: The Crossing Press, 1993.

Knight, Sirona. *Love, Sex, and Magick: Exploring the Spiritual Union Between Male and Female.* Secaucus, NJ: Citadel Press, 1999.

Kraig, Donald Michael, et al. *Modern Sex Magick.* St. Paul, MN: Llewellyn Publications, 1999.

Lapanja, Margie. *The Goddess' Guide to Love.* Berkeley, CA: Conari Press, 1999.

Lavabre, Marcel. *Aromatherapy Workbook.* Rochester, VT: Healing Arts Press, 1990.

Bibliography

Ravenwolf, Silver. *To Ride a Silver Broomstick.* St. Paul, MN: Llewellyn Publications, 1993.

Shehad, Margaret. *Gritman Guide to Essential Oils.* Friendswood, TX: Gritman Corporation, 1999.

Stassinopoulos, Agapi. *Conversations with the Goddesses.* New York, NY: Stewart, Tabori & Chang, 1999.

Stewart, R.J. *Celtic Gods Celtic Goddesses.* London, UK: Blandford, 1990.

Stoppard, Miriam. *The Magic of Sex.* New York, NY: DK Publishing, Inc., 1991.

Triple Image Films/Healing Arts Publishing. *The Secrets of Sacred Sex.* Healing Arts Publishing, 1994

Tye, Jeffery. "The Lingam Massage." Tantra.org, 1995.

Tye, Jeffery. "The Yoni Massage." Tantra.org, 1995.

Index